DISABILITY AND THE DISABLED – ISSUES, LAWS AND PROGRAMS

INDIVIDUALS WITH DISABILITIES

EDUCATION, EMPLOYMENT AND REHABILITATION

Disability and the Disabled – Issues, Laws and Programs

Additional books and e-books in this series can be found on Nova's website under the Series tab.

DISABILITY AND THE DISABLED – ISSUES, LAWS AND PROGRAMS

INDIVIDUALS WITH DISABILITIES

EDUCATION, EMPLOYMENT AND REHABILITATION

ASTON DELGADO
EDITOR

snova
New York

Additional color graphics may be available in the e-book version of this book.

Library of Congress Cataloging-in-Publication Data

ISBN: 978-1-53615-030-8

Published by Nova Science Publishers, Inc. † New York

CONTENTS

PREFACE

Since the enactment of P.L. 94-142, the predecessor legislation to the Individuals with Disabilities Education Act (IDEA), in 1975, the federal government has played a prominent role in encouraging the principle of educational equality for children with disabilities through a permanent, broad-scale federal assistance program. The IDEA is a grants statute that provides federal funding for the education of children with disabilities and requires, as a condition for the receipt of such funds, that states agree to provide a free appropriate public education (FAPE; i.e., specially designed instruction provided at no cost to the parents that meets the needs of a child with a disability) to every eligible child.

The transition from high school to the workforce can be a challenging time for students, and particularly for those with disabilities who may need additional services or guidance to achieve their goals. Studies have found that some employers are reluctant to hire people with disabilities, due, for example, to their perceptions about the costs of accommodations or the work capacity of people with disabilities. Studies have also found that many individuals with significant disabilities have been employed in sheltered workshops, where they are segregated from other employees and may be paid less than minimum wage.

Chapter 1 - Since the enactment of P.L. 94-142, the predecessor legislation to the Individuals with Disabilities Education Act (IDEA), in

1975, the federal government has played a prominent role in encouraging the principle of educational equality for children with disabilities through a permanent, broad-scale federal assistance program. The IDEA is a grants statute that provides federal funding for the education of children with disabilities and requires, as a condition for the receipt of such funds, that states agree to provide a free appropriate public education (FAPE; i.e., specially designed instruction provided at no cost to the parents that meets the needs of a child with a disability) to every eligible child. The IDEA, most recently reauthorized by P.L. 108-446 in 2004, was appropriated approximately $13.4 billion in FY2018. The largest part of the IDEA is Part B, Assistance for Education of all Children with Disabilities, which covers special education for children and youth with disabilities between the ages of 3 and 21. Approximately 92% of total IDEA appropriations fund the Part B, Section 611, grants-to-states program. Part B was funded at $12.7 billion in FY2018; and in the 2016-2017 school year, 6.8 million children ages 3 through 21 received educational services under it. In addition to the Part B grants-to-states program, the IDEA contains two programs for young children with disabilities. Part C authorizes federal funding for early intervention services to infants and toddlers with disabilities ages birth to three years, and Part B, Section 619 authorizes supplementary grants to states for preschool programs serving children with disabilities ages three to five. Each IDEA program serving children and youth with disabilities has followed a similar funding pattern. Appropriations for IDEA, Part B (Sections 611 and 619) and Part C increased steadily from each program's inception until the early 2000s. Since the IDEA's most recent reauthorization in FY2004, the funding for both Part B and Part C programs has fluctuated. The IDEA has two formulas for determining Part B grants to states: one for years when the appropriated amount available to states is greater than or equal to the amount available to states in the previous year, and one for years when the amount available to states is less than the amount available to states the previous year. In years when the appropriated amount for Part B increases or remains the same, each state receives its base-year (FY1999) grant amount plus a share of the "new money" (i.e., the amount above the FY1999 appropriation), based on the state's share of the national child population and national population of children living in poverty, adjusted according to one maximum and three minimum grant calculations, and ratably reduced when necessary. In years when the appropriated amount for Part B decreases, each state receives its base-year grant amount plus a share of the new money the state received the previous year, which has been ratably reduced proportional to the total new money available for the current year. This chapter will examine the development of the allocation formula for the Part B grants-to-states program, the major changes to the formula over the past 40 years, current funding levels and trends, and how allocations are currently calculated. Issues concerning the funding of special education and related services will also be discussed.

Chapter 2 - The Individuals with Disabilities Education Act (IDEA) is a statute that authorizes grant programs that support special education services. Under the IDEA, a series of conditions are attached to the receipt of grant funds. These conditions aim to provide certain educational and procedural guarantees for students with disabilities and their families. The grant programs authorized under the IDEA provide federal funding for special education and early intervention services for children with disabilities (birth to 21 years old) and require, as a condition for the receipt of such funds, the provision of a free appropriate public education (FAPE) (i.e., specially designed instruction provided at no cost to parents that meets the needs of a child with a disability) and an accessible early intervention system (a statewide system to provide and coordinate early intervention services for infants and toddlers with disabilities and their families). The IDEA also outlines and requires the use of procedural safeguards pertaining to the identification, evaluation, and placement of students in special education services that are intended to protect the rights of parents and children with disabilities. These procedures include parental rights to resolve disputes through a mediation process, and present and resolve complaints through a due process complaint procedure and through state complaint procedures. In the 2015-2016 school year, 6.8 million children ages 3 through 21 received educational services under Part B of the IDEA. To be covered under IDEA, a child with a disability must meet the categorical definition of disability in the act, and the child must require special education and related services as a result of the disability in order to benefit from public education. Once a child meets IDEA's eligibility criteria, FAPE is implemented through the Individualized Education Program (IEP), which is the plan for providing special education and related services by the local educational agency (LEA). The IEP is developed by an IEP team composed of school personnel and the child's parents or guardian. IDEA requires that children with disabilities be educated in the least restrictive environment. That is, to the maximum extent appropriate they are to be educated with children who are not disabled. In the fall of 2015, approximately 63% of all school-aged children with disabilities served by IDEA spent 80% or more of their time in a regular classroom. To implement IDEA, states and other entities (i.e., the District of Columbia, Puerto Rico, the Bureau of Indian Education, the outlying areas, and the freely associated states) receive grants based on a statutory formula. In FY2017, $13.05 billion was appropriated for IDEA. Most of the federal funds received by states are passed on to LEAs based on a statutory formula. IDEA also contains state and local maintenance of effort (MOE) requirements and supplement, not supplant (SNS) requirements aimed at increasing overall educational spending, rather than substituting federal funds for education spending at the state and local levels. Originally enacted in 1975, IDEA has been the subject of numerous reauthorizations to extend services and rights to children with disabilities. The most recent reauthorization of IDEA was P.L. 108-446, enacted in 2004. Funding for Part B, Assistance for Education of all Children with Disabilities, the largest and most often discussed part of the act, is permanently authorized. Funding for Part C, Infants and Toddlers with Disabilities, and Part D, National Activities, was authorized through FY2011. Funding for the programs continues to be authorized through annual appropriations.

Chapter 3 - The Individuals with Disabilities Education Act (IDEA) is a statute that authorizes grant programs that support special education services. Under the IDEA, a series of conditions are attached to the receipt of grant funds. These conditions aim to provide certain educational and procedural guarantees for students with disabilities and their families. The grant programs authorized under the IDEA provide federal funding for special education and early intervention services for children with disabilities (birth to 21 years old) and require, as a condition for the receipt of such funds, the provision of a free appropriate public education (FAPE) (i.e., specially designed instruction provided at no cost to parents that meets the needs of a child with a disability) and an accessible early intervention system (a statewide system to provide and coordinate early intervention services for infants and toddlers with disabilities and their families). The IDEA also outlines and requires the use of procedural safeguards pertaining to the identification, evaluation, and placement of students in special education services that are intended to protect the rights of parents and children with disabilities. These procedures include parental rights to resolve disputes through a mediation process, and present and resolve complaints through a due process complaint procedure and through state complaint procedures. Originally enacted in 1975, the IDEA has been the subject of numerous reauthorizations to extend services and rights to children with disabilities. The most recent reauthorization of the IDEA was P.L. 108-446, enacted in 2004. The 1986 reauthorization of the IDEA created a grants program that would provide early intervention services for infants and toddlers with disabilities and their families, what is now known as Part C, Infants and Toddlers with Disabilities. Funding for Part B of the IDEA, Assistance for Education of all Children with Disabilities, the largest part of the act, is permanently authorized. Funding for Part C, Infants and Toddlers with Disabilities, and Part D, National Activities, was authorized through FY2011. Funding for Part C and Part D programs continues to be authorized through annual appropriations. Part C of the IDEA authorizes a grant program to aid each state in implementing a system of early intervention services for infants and toddlers with disabilities and their families. In 2016, approximately 373,000 infants and toddlers between birth and three years old received early intervention services under Part C of the IDEA. Annual funding to each state for Part C programs is based upon the state's proportion of the number of children, birth through two years old, in the general population. In FY2018, approximately $13.4 billion was appropriated for the IDEA, $470 million of which was appropriated for Part C, representing 3.5% of total IDEA funding. Part C requires each state to implement a public awareness program and Child Find activities to identify infants and toddlers who may be eligible for early intervention services. To be eligible for early intervention services under Part C of the IDEA, an infant or toddler must meet his or her state's definition of an infant or toddler with a disability or developmental delay. Once a child meets the IDEA's eligibility criteria, the early intervention system provides an assessment of the needs of both the child and the child's family. Early intervention coordinators then either help the family coordinate services for their child through outside service providers or directly provide early intervention services to the child and the child's family, depending on the design of the early intervention system in the state. Before a child receiving Part C services turns three years old, the child is assessed to determine whether he or she will continue receiving IDEA services, and, if so, whether the child will remain in an extended Part C service arrangement or transition into a special education preschool program funded by Section 619 of Part B of the IDEA.

Chapter 4 - WIOA requires states to reserve at least 15 percent of their total State Vocational Rehabilitation Services program funds to provide pre-employment transition services to help students with disabilities transition from school to work. GAO was asked to review how states were implementing these services. This chapter examines (1) steps states reported taking to implement preemployment transition services, and (2) implementation challenges states reported and how Education has addressed them. GAO reviewed documents and funding data from Education, and federal laws and regulations; surveyed all 79 state VR agencies (74 responded); held discussion groups with representatives of 29 state VR agencies; and interviewed officials from Education and three states (Idaho, Illinois, and Maryland) GAO selected for variety in size and type of agencies, among other factors.

Chapter 5 - The Fair Labor Standards Act (FLSA), as amended, sets the minimum wage for covered workers at $7.25 per hour. Section 14(c) of the FLSA permits certified employers to pay a worker with a disability that impairs the worker's productive capacity a special minimum wage (SMW). The SMW may be below the federal minimum wage but must be commensurate with the worker's productivity and the job's prevailing wage. This chapter answers common questions related to SMWs. It covers

- federal legislation that authorizes SMWs;
- how individuals qualify for SMWs;
- how employers are certified to pay SMWs and how wage levels are set;
- data on employers that pay SMWs; and
- services that must be provided in conjunction with the payment of SMWs.

Chapter 6 - The VR program, administered by Education and state VR agencies, helps people with disabilities obtain employment. In 2014, WIOA made changes to the VR program, increasing its focus on serving employers, promoting career advancement as part of the broader goal of mainstream employment, and coordinating with other workforce programs. GAO was asked to review the VR program under WIOA. This chapter examines (1) the steps VR agencies have taken under WIOA to work with employers and place individuals in mainstream employment, and the extent Education has addressed any challenges; (2) how VR agencies have coordinated with other workforce programs and the extent federal agencies have addressed any challenges; and (3) how federal agencies have measured state VR agencies' efforts to serve employers. GAO surveyed all 79 VR agencies (74 responded); conducted three discussion groups with 36 state VR officials and four with 29 employers that worked with VR; interviewed VR and other workforce officials in three states, selected for geographic dispersion, among other factors; and reviewed relevant federal laws, regulations, and guidance.

In: Individuals with Disabilities
Editor: Aston Delgado
ISBN: 978-1-53615-030-8

Chapter 1

THE INDIVIDUALS WITH DISABILITIES EDUCATION ACT (IDEA) FUNDING: A PRIMER*

Kyrie E. Dragoo

SUMMARY

Since the enactment of P.L. 94-142, the predecessor legislation to the Individuals with Disabilities Education Act (IDEA), in 1975, the federal government has played a prominent role in encouraging the principle of educational equality for children with disabilities through a permanent, broad-scale federal assistance program. The IDEA is a grants statute that provides federal funding for the education of children with disabilities and requires, as a condition for the receipt of such funds, that states agree to provide a free appropriate public education (FAPE; i.e., specially designed instruction provided at no cost to the parents that meets the needs of a child with a disability) to every eligible child.

The IDEA, most recently reauthorized by P.L. 108-446 in 2004, was appropriated approximately $13.4 billion in FY2018. The largest part of the IDEA is Part B, Assistance for Education of all Children with Disabilities, which covers special education for children and youth with

* This is an edited, reformatted and augmented version of Congressional Research Service Publication No. R44624, updated October 1, 2018.

disabilities between the ages of 3 and 21. Approximately 92% of total IDEA appropriations fund the Part B, Section 611, grants-to-states program. Part B was funded at $12.7 billion in FY2018; and in the 2016-2017 school year, 6.8 million children ages 3 through 21 received educational services under it. In addition to the Part B grants-to-states program, the IDEA contains two programs for young children with disabilities. Part C authorizes federal funding for early intervention services to infants and toddlers with disabilities ages birth to three years, and Part B, Section 619 authorizes supplementary grants to states for preschool programs serving children with disabilities ages three to five. Each IDEA program serving children and youth with disabilities has followed a similar funding pattern. Appropriations for IDEA, Part B (Sections 611 and 619) and Part C increased steadily from each program's inception until the early 2000s. Since the IDEA's most recent reauthorization in FY2004, the funding for both Part B and Part C programs has fluctuated. The IDEA has two formulas for determining Part B grants to states: one for years when the appropriated amount available to states is greater than or equal to the amount available to states in the previous year, and one for years when the amount available to states is less than the amount available to states the previous year. In years when the appropriated amount for Part B increases or remains the same, each state receives its base-year (FY1999) grant amount plus a share of the "new money" (i.e., the amount above the FY1999 appropriation), based on the state's share of the national child population and national population of children living in poverty, adjusted according to one maximum and three minimum grant calculations, and ratably reduced when necessary. In years when the appropriated amount for Part B decreases, each state receives its base-year grant amount plus a share of the new money the state received the previous year, which has been ratably reduced proportional to the total new money available for the current year.

This chapter will examine the development of the allocation formula for the Part B grants-to-states program, the major changes to the formula over the past 40 years, current funding levels and trends, and how allocations are currently calculated. Issues concerning the funding of special education and related services will also be discussed.

INTRODUCTION TO THE IDEA

The Individuals with Disabilities Education Act (IDEA)[1] provides federal funding for the education of children with disabilities and requires,

---

[1] 20 U.S.C. §1400 et seq.; P.L. 108-446.

as a condition for the receipt of such funds, the provision of a free appropriate public education (FAPE) for children with disabilities. The IDEA's predecessor legislation, the Education for All Handicapped Children Act (P.L. 94-142, passed in 1975), responded to increased awareness of the need to educate children with disabilities, and to judicial decisions requiring that states provide an education for children with disabilities if they provided an education for children without disabilities.[2]

In its current form, the IDEA both authorizes federal funding for special education and related services[3] and, for states that accept these funds,[4] sets out principles under which special education and related services are to be provided. Over the past four decades, the IDEA has been the subject of numerous reauthorizations to extend services and rights to children with disabilities. The most recent reauthorization was P.L. 108-446 in 2004.[5] Funding for IDEA Part B, Assistance for Education of all Children with Disabilities, is permanently authorized.[6] Funding for Part C, Infants and Toddlers with Disabilities, and Part D, National Activities, was authorized through FY2011.[7] Funding for the programs continues to be authorized through annual appropriations.

---

[2] For a more detailed discussion of the congressional intent behind the enactment of predecessor legislation to the IDEA, the Education of All Handicapped Children Act, P.L. 94-142, congressional clients may request archived CRS Report 95-669, *The Individuals with Disabilities Education Act: Congressional Intent*.

[3] Related services (e.g., assistive technology or physical therapy) assist children with disabilities to help them benefit from special education (20 U.S.C. §1401(26); P.L. 108-446 §602(26)).

[4] Currently, all states receive IDEA funding. The IDEA defines the term "State" as "each of the 50 States, the District of Columbia, the Commonwealth of Puerto Rico, and each of the outlying areas," P.L. 108-446, §602 (31).

[5] For a discussion of the 2004 amendments made by P.L. 108-446, congressional clients may request archived CRS Report RL32716, *Individuals with Disabilities Education Act (IDEA): Analysis of Changes Made by* P.L. 108-446. For an overview of the IDEA regulations from the Department of Education, congressional clients may request archived CRS Report RL33649, *The Individuals with Disabilities Education Act (IDEA): Final Regulations for* P.L. 108-446; and CRS Report R40055, *The Individuals with Disabilities Education Act: Final Part B Regulations*.

[6] For more information on Part B of the IDEA, see CRS Report R41833, *The Individuals with Disabilities Education Act (IDEA), Part B: Key Statutory and Regulatory Provisions*.

[7] IDEA authorizes appropriations for Part C and Part D programs and activities through FY2010. These authorities were automatically extended for an additional fiscal year by the General Education Provisions Act (GEPA; 20 U.S.C.§1226a). For more information on Part C of the IDEA, see CRS Report R43631, *The Individuals with Disabilities Education Act (IDEA), Part C: Early Intervention for Infants and Toddlers with Disabilities*.

Table 1. Structure and Funding of the IDEA (Funding in thousands of dollars)

IDEA Part	Description	FY2018 Funding	Percentage of Total IDEA Funding
Part A—General Provisions	Includes findings, purposes, and definitions	—	—
Part B—Assistance for Education of all Children with Disabilities	Contains provisions relating to the education of school aged children and authorizes the grants- to-states program (Section 611) and state grants program for preschool children with disabilities (Section 619)		
	Section 611, Grants to States	$12,277,848	92.0%
	Section 619, Preschool Grants	$381,120	2.9%
	Subtotal, Part B	$12,658,968	94.8%
Part C—Infants and Toddlers with Disabilities	Authorizes state grants for programs serving infants and toddlers with disabilities	$470,000	3.5%
Part D—National Activities to Improve Education of Children with Disabilities	Contains the requirements for and authorizes various national activities	$222,133	1.7%
IDEA Total		$13,351,101	100%

Source: Table prepared by CRS based on a review of the IDEA. Funding amounts are from Department of Education budget tables for FY2018, https://www2.ed.gov/about/overview/budget/budget18/18action.pdf.

The Structure and Funding of the IDEA

The IDEA consists of four parts. Part A contains the general provisions, including the purposes of the act and definitions. Part B contains provisions relating to the education of school aged children (the grants-to-states program) and the state grants program for preschool children with disabilities (Section 619). Part C authorizes state grants for programs serving infants and toddlers with disabilities. Part D contains the requirements for various national activities designed to improve the education of children with disabilities. Table 1 shows the structure and funding of the IDEA and is followed by a more detailed discussion of the four parts of the act.

Part A: General Provisions

Part A includes congressional findings pertinent to the act, the purposes of the act, and definitions. The definitions included in Part A are important in interpreting the requirements of the act.

These include, among others, definitions of child with a disability, specific learning disability, free appropriate public education, individualized education program, local educational agency, related services, special education, supplementary aids and services, transition services, and excess costs.

Part B: Assistance for Education of All Children with Disabilities

Part B provides federal funding to states for the education of children with disabilities and requires, as a condition for the receipt of such funds, the provision of a FAPE to children with disabilities between the ages of 3 and 21.[8] School districts within participating states must identify, locate, and evaluate all children with disabilities, regardless of the severity of their disability, to determine which children are eligible for special education and related services. Each child receiving services must have an Individualized Education Program (IEP), created by an IEP team, delineating the specific special education and related services to be provided to meet his or her needs. The statute also contains procedural safeguards, which are provisions to protect the rights of parents and children with disabilities to ensure the provision of FAPE. Section 619 authorizes grants to states for preschool programs serving children with disabilities ages three to five. Section 619 is a relatively brief section of the law and deals mostly with the state and

---

[8] Currently 18 states, the District of Columbia, and Puerto Rico provide children a free appropriate public education until the age of 21, the remaining states stop providing FAPE to students at 18, 19, or 20 years of age. The population used in IDEA formula calculations is based on the age range served in each state. A list of the age ranges served in each state can be found in *Table A-1* in *Appendix A* of this chapter.

substate funding formulas for the preschool program grants and state-level activities.

Part C: Infants and Toddlers with Disabilities

The general purpose of Part C is to aid each state in creating and maintaining "a statewide, comprehensive, coordinated, multidisciplinary, interagency system that provides early intervention services for infants and toddlers with disabilities and their families."[9] Services focus on children (and their families) from birth through age two who are experiencing or have a high probability of experiencing "developmental delay" (as defined by the state) with respect to physical, mental, or other capacities.[10] Services are detailed for each child and his or her family in an Individualized Family Service Plan (IFSP). To the maximum extent feasible, services are to be provided in "natural environments," including the home, with other infants and toddlers who are not disabled. States are required to identify a state lead agency, which might be the state educational agency (SEA) but could be other state agencies, to coordinate the system.

Part D: National Activities to Improve Education of Children with Disabilities[11]

Part D authorizes competitive grants to improve the education of children with disabilities under three subparts with different areas of emphasis: (1) state personnel development; (2) personnel preparation, technical assistance, model demonstration projects, and dissemination of information; and (3) support to improve results for children.

---

[9] U.S.C. §1431(b)(1); P.L. 108-446 §631(b)(1).

[10] Under certain circumstances, children with disabilities age three and over may continue to receive Part C early intervention services until they are eligible to enter kindergarten; 20 U.S.C. §14345(c); P.L. 108-446 §635(c).

[11] In addition to the statutory provisions in Part D, see the following for more information on these activities: U.S. Department of Education, *Fiscal Year 2019, Budget Summary*, pp. 19-21; and U.S. Department of Education, *Guide to U.S. Department of Education Programs, 2010*, pp. 254-262.

- Under Subpart 1, competitive grants are made to SEAs for state personnel development grants to assist SEAs "in reforming and improving their systems for personnel preparation and professional development in early intervention, educational, and transitions services." Under these grants, personnel preparation and development may be provided for special education teachers, regular education [12]teachers, principals, administrators, related services personnel, paraprofessionals, and early intervention personnel serving infants, toddlers, preschoolers, or children with disabilities.
- Under Subpart 2, competitive grants are made to entities such as SEAs, local education agencies (LEAs),[13] institutions of higher education (IHEs), and nonprofit organizations for personnel development to help ensure that there are adequate numbers of personnel with skills and knowledge needed to help children with disabilities succeed,[14] for technical assistance and dissemination of material based on knowledge gained through research and practice,[15] and for studies and evaluations.[16]
- Under Subpart 3, competitive grants are made to nonprofit organizations for parent training and information centers, which provide parents of children with disabilities with needed training and information to work with professionals in meeting the early intervention and special education needs of their children.[17] Competitive grants are also made to entities such as SEAs, LEAs, IHEs, and nonprofit organizations for research, development, and

[12] 20 U.S.C. §1451(a); P.L. 108-446 §651(a).

[13] The term "local educational agency" means "a public board of education or other public authority legally constituted within a state for either administrative control or direction of, or to perform a service function for, public elementary schools or secondary schools in a city, county, township, school district, or other political subdivision of a state, or for such combination of school districts or counties as are recognized in a state as an administrative agency for its public elementary schools or secondary schools." 20 U.S.C. §14011(19); P.L. 108-446 §601(19). The term "school district" is often used instead of local educational agency.

[14] 20 U.S.C. §1462; P.L. 108-446 §662

[15] 20 U.S.C. §1463; P.L. 108-446 §663.

[16] 20 U.S.C. §1464; P.L. 108-446 §664.

[17] 20 U.S.C. §§1471, 1472, 1473; P.L. 108-446 §§671, 672, 673.

other activities that promote the use of technology in providing special education and early intervention services.[18]

Current IDEA Funding

Part B is the largest part of the IDEA, and it received nearly 95%, $12.7 billion, of the act's total funding in FY2018. Part B's funding is authorized in two different sections. Section 611, which covers children between the ages of 3 and 21 receiving special education and related services in public schools,[19] received $12.3 billion in FY2018. Section 619, which provides supplementary preschool grants for children between the ages of 3 and 5, received $381.1 million in FY2018.

In comparison, as is shown in *Table 1*, Part C was appropriated $470 million (3.5% of IDEA funding) in FY2018. Less than 2% of the total IDEA funding went to Part D.

IDEA Funding Trends

The IDEA is one of the largest educational programs overseen by the U.S. Department of Education (ED). As *Figure 1* displays, from the first year of funding in 1977 until about a decade ago, appropriations for the Part B grants-to-states program[20] had been rising rapidly. In the first 20 years of funding for the Part B program, appropriations increased approximately 470% in constant 2017 dollars. Between the last two reauthorizations of the IDEA in 1997 and 2004, Part B appropriations rose an average of 18% per year in constant dollars. However, Part B funding trends changed after the 2004 reauthorization, and appropriations have fluctuated in the years since.

---

[18] 20 U.S.C. §1474; P.L. 108-446 §674.

[19] The age range provided a FAPE varies by state and likewise the age range in the funding formula varies according to state policies. See footnote 42 for more information.

[20] For further information, see CRS Report R41833, The Individuals with Disabilities Education Act (IDEA), Part B: Key Statutory and Regulatory Provisions.

Part B funding reached its highest levels in FY2005 and FY2009,[21] with inflation-adjusted amounts exceeding $13.1 billion each year. In FY2017 the appropriation was $12 billion, and in FY2018 it was $12.3 billion.

Despite recent fluctuations in Part B appropriations, funding for the Part B grants-to-states program increased steadily for most of its first four decades (*Figure 1*). In contrast, funding levels for the two early childhood grant programs, after experiencing substantial growth in earlier periods in program history, have declined in constant dollar amounts in more recent periods.

The Part B, Section 619 preschool grants program began with a period of relatively low funding between FY1980 and FY1986 ($25 million to $29 million), followed by a period of rapid escalation in funding between FY1987 ($180 million) and FY1995 ($360 million). The year-to-year escalation in Section 619 funding slowed over the next five years. In FY2000, Section 619 funding reached its highest annual appropriation level in actual dollars ($390 million), and it maintained that appropriation for the next two years. From FY2003 through the present, Section 619 appropriations have fluctuated somewhat in actual dollars and declined in constant dollars. The Section 619 preschool grants program received its highest level of funding in constant FY2017 dollars in FY1995 ($578 million). In FY2018, the Part B, Section 619 preschool grants program was appropriated $381 million.

The Part C, infants and families program experienced a period of relatively constant funding growth for its first 15 years; Part C appropriations increased from $50 million in FY1987 to over $444 million in FY2004. In the years since, the IDEA Part C grants program has received relatively level appropriations in actual dollars and declining funding in constant 2017 dollars. Between FY2004, the year of the IDEA's most recent reauthorization, and FY2012, funding in nominal dollars for the Part C program changed relatively little from one year to the next, while funding in

---

[21] The FY2009 amount refers only to regular appropriations; additional IDEA funding provided by the American Recovery and Reinvestment Act (ARRA, P.L. 111-5) is not considered. Including the $11.3 billion in ARRA funds, the amount appropriated in FY2009 was $22.8 billion in nominal dollars, or $26 billion in FY2017 constant dollars.

inflation-adjusted dollars eroded. For the past five years, appropriations for the Part C program have fluctuated. In FY2018, the Part C, infants and families program was appropriated $470 million.

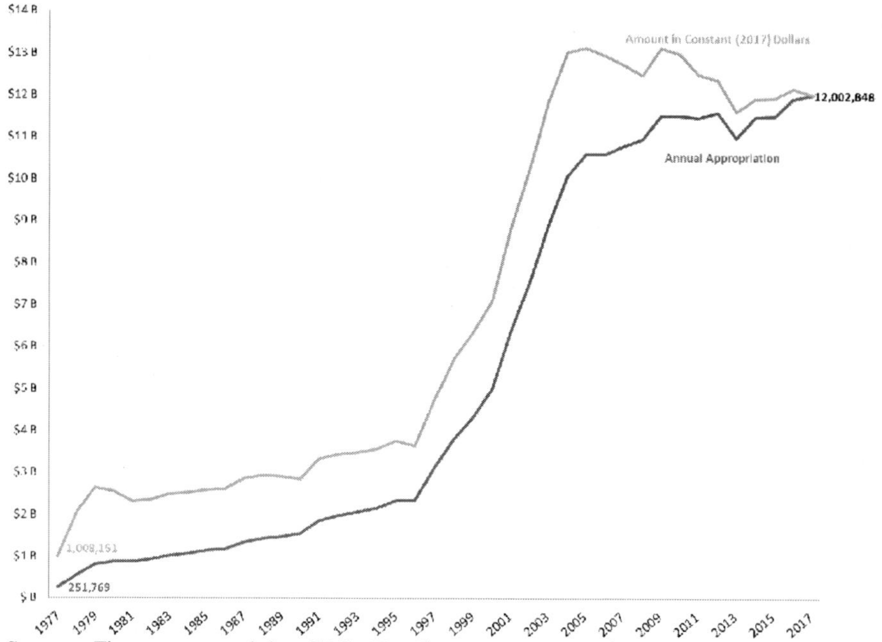

Source: Figure prepared by CRS. Funding amounts are from U.S. Department of Education budget tables, https://www2.ed.gov/about/overview/budget/tables.html.

Notes: Constant dollar amounts show inflation-adjusted funding amounts calculated using the Consumer Price Index-All Urban Consumers (CPI-U).

The funding amount for FY2009 only displays regular appropriations; additional IDEA funding provided by the American Recovery and Reinvestment Act (ARRA, P.L. 111-5) is not displayed.

Figure 1. IDEA, Part B, Grants to States Funding, FY1977-FY2017 (Funding in billions, shown in actual and constant FY2017 dollars)

The Part C, infants and families program experienced a period of relatively constant funding growth for its first 15 years; Part C appropriations increased from $50 million in FY1987 to over $444 million in FY2004. In the years since, the IDEA Part C grants program has received relatively level appropriations in actual dollars and declining funding in constant 2017 dollars. Between FY2004, the year of the IDEA's most recent reauthorization, and FY2012, funding in nominal dollars for the Part C program changed relatively little from one year to the next, while funding in inflation-adjusted dollars eroded. For the past five years, appropriations for the Part C program have fluctuated. In FY2018, the Part C, infants and families program was appropriated $470 million.

HISTORICAL REVIEW OF FUNDING PROVISIONS IN THE IDEA AND RELATED ACTS

Federal laws concerning children with disabilities date from the early 19th century, but it was not until the Elementary and Secondary Education Act (ESEA) was reauthorized for the first time in 1966 that the first general federal assistance was provided to states for the education of children with disabilities. The original version of the ESEA, which Congress enacted in 1965 as P.L. 89- 10, did not specify assistance for children with disabilities. However, the Senate Committee on Labor and Public Welfare report on the legislation included a provision stating that upon a U.S. Office of Education determination of disability, children with disabilities would be considered "educationally deprived" for purposes of eligibility for the ESEA Title I compensatory education program for disadvantaged children.

P.L. 89-750, the Elementary and Secondary Education Act Amendments of 1966, established a new Title VI of the ESEA, separately authorizing an assistance program for projects in states to educate children with disabilities. Sponsors of this law argued that the U.S. Office of Education had not appropriately responded to the needs of children with disabilities under the ESEA Title I program. P.L. 89-750 authorized a two-year program of project grants to states for the education of children with disabilities at the preschool, elementary, and secondary school levels.[22] Allotments of grant funds to states were based on the state's population of children with disabilities ages 3 through 21 in need of special education and related

[22] The authorization of appropriations for Title VI under P.L. 89-750 was $50 million for FY1967 and $150 million for FY1968.

services.[23] P.L. 89-750 also authorized a National Advisory Committee on the Education of the Handicapped, and established a bureau within the Office of Education to administer programs for the education and training of children and youth with disabilities.

The Education of the Handicapped Act (EHA)

The ESEA Amendments of 1970 (P.L. 91-230) repealed Title VI and created a separate law, the Education of the Handicapped Act (EHA), to consolidate all federal educational assistance for children with disabilities into one statute. The new program of assistance to states was essentially a grant program that supported projects providing services for students with disabilities, which was authorized for three fiscal years.[24]

By 1970, some Members of Congress argued that greater emphasis should be placed on EHA assistance to states because of the number of school-age children with disabilities who reportedly were unserved by states. The House Committee on Education and Labor report on the bill that would become P.L. 91-230 noted that by U.S. Office of Education estimates, 60% of the total school-age population of children with disabilities in the United States were not receiving special education services.[25] The committee did not recommend any changes in the federal program of project grants to states to address the problem, but it urged full program funding. The committee noted that the history of assistance programs for children with disabilities had been "marked by serious discrepancies between

[23] A limited number of disabilities covered by the IDEA were considered qualifying conditions for the receipt of special education and related services under P.L. 89-750. Of the 14 categories of disabilities currently included in the IDEA regulations, eight were listed in P.L. 89-750. In current terminology, the categories in P.L. 89-750 were intellectual disability, hearing impairment, deafness, speech or language impairment, emotional disturbance, orthopedic impairment, other health impairment, and visual impairment including blindness.

[24] The EHA program of assistance to states was authorized for three fiscal years at the following levels: $200 million for FY1971; $210 million for FY1972; and $220 million for FY1973.

[25] U.S. Congress, House Committee on Education and Labor, Elementary and Secondary Amendments of 1969, Report to accompany H.R. 514, 91st Cong., 1st session, Report. No. 91-114, Washington, DC, U.S. GPO, 1969, p. 5.

authorizations and appropriations." In FY1969, for example, appropriations were only about 18% of the authorization.

By 1974, when the EHA state grant program was next reauthorized in P.L. 93-380, Congress had become increasingly persuaded that the program did not adequately address the educational needs of children with disabilities. States, under court mandates and their own laws, had major new responsibilities to provide educational services to all children with disabilities, but due to financial constraints many were unable to meet minimum educational requirements. The amendments enacted in P.L. 93-380 that provided a one-year "emergency" program of assistance to states set the stage for the enactment of the IDEA's predecessor legislation—the Education of All Handicapped Children Act (P.L. 94-142)—in 1975.

Education for All Handicapped Children Act

As early as 1972, an Education for All Handicapped Children Act was proposed in the 92nd Congress in S. 3614, introduced by Senator Harrison Williams, Chairman of the Senate Committee on Labor and Public Welfare, and in H.R. 15727, introduced by Representative John Brademas, Chairman of the House Subcommittee on Select Education.[26] These basically similar bills would have authorized federal assistance to states to help them implement the Supreme Court's mandate that all children with disabilities receive appropriate educational services. In contrast to the existing federal program of grants supporting projects, the program authorized by these bills would have provided federal payments to states for up to 75% of the excess costs incurred by school districts for educating children with disabilities.

In his statement introducing S. 3614 Senator Williams noted:

> We have increased Federal assistance [for children with disabilities] from $45 million 5 years ago to $215 million in the present fiscal year. But

[26] Congressional Research Service No. 86-552 EPW, P.L. 94-142, *The Education for All Handicapped Children Act: Its development, implementation, and current issues*, by C. J. Fraas, February 10, 1986. (Archived, available to congressional clients on request.)

> these have been token expenditures. Nowhere in our public laws or in our budget figures do we find acceptance for the proposition that all handicapped children have the right to an education. It has been the courts which have forced us to the realization that we can delay no longer in making just such a commitment.
>
> [W]e at the Federal level are going to have to change our traditional methods of investing money. The theory that the Federal Government can provide minimal assistance to the states as incentive grants to provide extensive educational services simply does not meet the mark in this instance...It is hard to argue to the states that the Federal Government is serious about full educational opportunity for all handicapped children when we are not willing to invest money to make this goal a reality. If we are going to make a real commitment to full and appropriate services, and expect the states to carry through on this commitment, we will have to put our money where our mouth is.[27]

At the beginning of the 93rd Congress, Senator Williams and Representative Brademas reintroduced the Education for All Handicapped Children Act as S. 6 and H.R. 70, respectively. The Nixon Administration opposed the Williams and Brademas proposals, and the 93rd Congress ended without action on either bill.

The Education Amendments of 1974 (P.L. 93-380) included a significant change in the EHA state grant program. Offered by Senator Charles Mathias of Maryland, the "Mathias amendment" authorized a program of federal assistance to states, for FY1975 only, through a funding allotment equaling a state's population of children ages 3 through 21 multiplied by $8.75. This authorization represented a threefold increase in the amount last authorized for the state grant program under P.L. 91-230. The Mathias amendment also, for the first time, required states as a condition of receiving assistance to adopt certain program policies and due process procedures such as those that were being proposed in S. 6 and H.R. 70. When the Mathias amendment was considered, Senators agreed that it should be thought of as an interim emergency measure pending the enactment of S. 6,

---

[27] *Congressional Record*, v. 118, May 16, 1972, p. 17478.

which was being crafted by the Senate Committee on Labor and Public Welfare after extensive hearings and more thorough examination.[28]

P.L. 93-380 became law on August 24, 1974. Appropriations for FY1975 for the Mathias amendment were $100 million, approximately 15% of the amount that would have needed to be appropriated to fully fund the program, though twice the FY1974 appropriations for the state grant program. P.L. 93-554, the Supplemental Appropriations Act for Fiscal Year 1975, which provided the FY1975 appropriations for the EHA state grant program, provided an additional $100 million in appropriations for obligations under the program in FY1976.

The Education for All Handicapped Children Act was reintroduced in the 94th Congress by Senator Williams in the Senate and Representative Brademas in the House, each bill with over 20 cosponsors. In addition to the hearings held in the previous Congress, several more days of hearings were devoted to the measures in both the House and Senate in the spring of 1975.[29] The major concerns of witnesses before the Senate subcommittee involved the most appropriate formula for the distribution of funds under S. 6, and the best way to enforce the education rights of children with disabilities and measure compliance. Similarly, the House committee report included views of certain committee members focusing mainly on whether the authorization levels implied by the formula might be unrealistic.

Conference Action

The Senate and House appointed members to a conference committee to resolve their differing versions of the Education for All Handicapped Children Act. The conference committee met on five days in October 1975 and agreed to a compromise version of the bill on October 30. Some of the most significant differences between the Senate and House proposals related to funding issues, including the funding formula, within-state distribution of

---

[28] 28 Hubert Humphrey, Education Amendments of 1974, *Congressional Record*, v. 120, May 20, 1974, p. 15273.

[29] Senate Hearings: Education for all handicapped children, A75. Hearings, 94th Cong., 1st sess., on S. 6. April 8, 9, and 15, 1975, Washington, DC, U.S. GPO, 1975. House Hearings: Extension of Education of the Handicapped Act, Hearings, 94th Cong., 1st sess., on part X, April 9-10 and June 9, 1975, Washington, DC, U.S. GPO, 1975.

funds, the excess costs provisions, preschool incentive grants, and administrative and planning costs.

The conference committee agreed to a formula that would provide a maximum grant for each state that is equal to its count of children with disabilities served multiplied by a gradually increasing percentage of the national average per pupil expenditure (APPE)—beginning at 5% of the APPE in FY1978, increasing to 40% in FY1982, and then remaining at 40% every year thereafter. The authorization was permanent, and would become effective in FY1978.[30] The maximum allowable grant that each state could receive per special education student from FY1982 onward (i.e., 40% of the APPE) came to be known as the "full funding" amount for the Education of All Handicapped Children Act, and later for the IDEA. The funding states received in FY1977 was set as the base-year amount—no state could receive less than it had that year. In years when Congress did not appropriate enough to meet the authorized level of 40% of the APPE, each state's award was reduced proportionally.

The Senate Committee on Labor and Public Welfare explained its rationale for using states' special education child count in 1975, stating:

> The Committee wished to develop a formula which would target funding and eligibility for funding on the population of handicapped children for whom services would be provided. The Committee adopted this formula in order to provide an incentive to states to serve all handicapped children and to assure that the entitlement is based on the number of children actually receiving special education and related services within the State and for whom the State or the local educational agency is paying for such education. The formula in existing law, the Education of the Handicapped Act, distributes Federal funds to the States on the number of all children, aged three to twenty-one within such State.

[30] In the interim, the "Mathias amendment formula" would apply under the following limits on appropriations: $100 million for FY1976; "such sums as are necessary" for the transition period; and $200 million for FY1977. The federal fiscal year's end date changed in FY1976 from June 30 to September 30. The "transition period" was the three months between these dates and the beginning of FY1977 on October 1, 1976.

The Committee has developed a formula which generates funds on the basis of the handicapped children receiving an education within a State.[31]

President Ford Signs the Bill

President Gerald Ford signed S. 6 on November 29, 1975, and it became P.L. 94-142. In a statement on the approval of the bill, the President noted his reservations that the legislation falsely raised the hopes and expectations of the disabilities community because of excessive and unrealistic authorization levels. President Ford said, "Despite my strong support for full educational opportunities for our handicapped children, the funding levels proposed in this bill will simply not be possible if Federal expenditures are to be brought under control and a balanced budget achieved over the next few years."[32] In the four decades since the signing of the Education for All Handicapped Children Act, appropriations for the Part B grants-to-states program have never met the authorized "full-funding" level of 40% of the national APPE.

Funding Formula Changes: IDEA 1997

Since 1975, Congress has reauthorized the federal special education law five times, most recently in 2004. Known as the Individuals with Disabilities Education Act (IDEA) since its 1990 reauthorization, the act's funding provisions have undergone several changes over the past 40 years, the most significant of which were implemented in the 1997 reauthorization.[33]

In an effort to ensure that states would identify and serve all children in need of special education services, Congress designed P.L. 94-142's funding formula to reward states for identifying students with disabilities for special education services and for continuing to provide them with special education

---

[31] U. S. Congress, Senate Committee on Labor and Public Welfare, Education of the Handicapped Act as Amended Through December 31, 1975, Report No. 72-611, June 2, 1975, Washington, DC: U.S. GPO, pp. 204-205.

[32] Education for All Handicapped Children Act of 1975, Weekly Compilation of Presidential Documents, v. 11, no. 9, p. 1335.

[33] P.L. 105-17.

once they were identified. Congress encouraged states to serve all children in need of special education and related services by tying Part B funding to the number of special education students each state served.

By the mid-1990s, Congress found that their goal of ensuring public schools would identify and serve children with disabilities had been successful; however, a growing concern was a disproportionate number of minority children being identified as disabled, particularly in the more subjective disability categories of specific learning disability (SLD), intellectual disability, and emotional disturbance.[34] The committee reports accompanying the 1997 IDEA amendments presented Congress's concern about the disproportionate representation of minorities in special education and explained their rationale for a new state allocation formula.[35] The House Report of the Committee on Education and the Workforce[36] stated:

> The Committee developed the change in formula to address the problem of over-identification of children with disabilities. When the Act was first passed in 1975, States were not providing educational services to many children with disabilities. Therefore, Congress proposed to distribute federal funds for special education services in order to encourage and reward States for serving eligible children. In the 22 years since then, the States have made excellent progress in identifying children with disabilities and providing them access to special education, and are now serving 5.5 million children with disabilities or approximately 10 percent of children aged 3 through 17. Logically, a formula was established at that time that based funding on counting the number of children with disabilities identified. This was to encourage States to proactively locate children with disabilities.
>
> Today, the growing problem is over identifying children as disabled when they might not be truly disabled. The challenge today is not so much how to provide access to special education services but how to

[34] In 1997, the term "mental retardation" was used in place of "intellectual disability" and "serious emotional disturbance" was used instead of "emotional disturbance" (P.L. 105-17, §1401(3)). P.L. 108-446 used the term "emotional disturbance" without the word "serious" preceding it for the first time. P.L. 111-256, commonly referred to as Rosa's Law, required references to "mental retardation" in IDEA and other federal laws to be changed to "intellectual disability."

[35] H.Rept. 105-95. See also S.Rept. 105-17.

[36] H.Rept. 105-95 (Funding formula §611).

appropriately provide educational services to children with disabilities in order to improve educational results for such children. As States consider this issue, more and more States are exploring alternatives for serving more children with learning problems in the regular educational classroom. But in doing so, they face the prospect of reductions in Federal funds, as long as funding is tied to child counts.

While it is unlikely that individual educators ever identify children for the additional funding that such identification brings, the financial incentive reduces the proactive scrutiny that such referrals would receive if they did not have the additional monetary benefit. It also reduces the scrutiny of children who might be moved back out of special education. In-State funding formulas that follow the current disability-based Federal child-count formula further reduce such scrutiny, with more children being identified to draw additional State funds.

This problem is most intense with minority children, especially African-American males. Over-identification of minority children, particularly in urban schools with high proportions of minority students, remains a serious and growing problem in this Nation. The problem also contributes to the referral of minority special education students to more restrictive environments. The committee is also cognizant, however, that in some areas under identification remains a problem, particularly for minority children.

The report explained the change from a formula based on the number of children receiving special education to a formula based on the total population of children in each state and the percentage of those children living in poverty:

The Committee has squarely faced this problem by shifting, once the targeted threshold is reached, to a formula of which 85 percent of additional funds is based on the total school age population and 15 percent is based on the poverty statistic for children in a State. This system was encouraged in the 1994 report of the Department of Education's Inspector General. The Inspector General noted:'Because [a population-based] method [of allocating funds] uses objective data derived for other purposes, [this method] eliminates the financial incentives for manipulating student counts [that exist in the current formula], including retaining students in special education just to continue receiving Federal funds." The Committee added a poverty factor to the formula because there is a link between poverty and certain forms of disability. This concept was also encouraged by the Inspector General's report.

Based on the significant progress that has been made in providing access to special education and concerns about the over-identification of children as disabled, the Committee believes this new formula will address many of these concerns. This change will enable States to undertake good practices for addressing the learning needs of more children in the regular classroom without the unnecessary categorization or labeling thereby risking the loss of Federal funds. Changing the Federal formula may also motivate States to change their own formulas for distributing State aid in ways that eliminate inappropriate financial incentives for referring children to special education.

The funding formula adopted through the 1997 IDEA amendments was set to take effect the year the federal appropriation for the grants-to-states program first exceeded $4.9 billion. The formula guaranteed states a minimum base-year amount, which was set as the amount states received the year before the new formula took effect.[37] Since the IDEA appropriation exceeded $4.9 billion for the first time in FY2000, the base-year amount states were guaranteed was their FY1999 funding level.

In years when Congress appropriated more funding to the grants-to-states program than it had the year before, funding exceeding the base-year amount would be allocated to states based on the total population of children ages 3 through 21[38] in the state and the percentage of those children living in poverty. Of the funding over the base-year amount, 85% was awarded based on the population of children ages 3 through 21 in the state (not only children with disabilities), and the remaining 15% was based on the state's share of

[37] P.L. 105-17 §611(e)(1).

[38] Currently 18 states, the District of Columbia, and Puerto Rico provide children a free appropriate public education until the age of 21, the remaining states stop providing FAPE to students at 18, 19, or 20 years of age. The population used in IDEA formula calculations is based on the age range served in each state. A list of the age ranges served in each state can be found in *Table A-1* in *Appendix A* of this chapter.

children living in poverty. The full funding amount of 40% of the APPE was maintained in the formula adopted through the 1997 amendments. While there were changes and additions made to the IDEA formula in the 2004 reauthorization, which will be discussed in the next section of this chapter, the basic framework of the formula adopted through the 1997 amendments remains in place today.

PROCEDURES USED TO ALLOCATE IDEA FUNDS

Part B Grants to States

What follows is a description of grant allocation procedures authorized under current law. After the Secretary of Education (the Secretary) has reserved funds for technical assistance[39] and for payments to the outlying areas, the freely associated states, and the Secretary of the Interior[40] for a fiscal year, the Secretary allocates the remaining IDEA Part B amount among the states. Part B formula grants to states are calculated based on one of two scenarios: (1) the appropriated amount available to states for the current fiscal year is greater than or equal to the amount that was available to states in the previous year, or (2) the amount available to states in the current year is less than the amount available to states the previous year. *Figure 2* summarizes the process of determining state allocations whether appropriations increase, remain the same, or decrease. The following two sections of this chapter will examine how IDEA allocations are calculated in years when funding increases or remains the same, and in years when funding decreases.

---

[39] 34 C.F.R. §300.702.

[40] 34 C.F.R. §300.701. "The Secretary shall ... make payments to the Secretary of the Interior to be distributed to tribes, tribal organizations, or consortia of the above entities for the coordination of assistance in the provision of early intervention services by the States to infants and toddlers with disabilities and their families on reservations served by elementary schools and secondary schools for Indian children operated or funded by the Department of the Interior." P.L. 108-446 §643(b)(1).

Level or Increased Federal IDEA Part B Funding

The IDEA Part B provisions specifying the allocation procedures when Part B appropriations are the same as or greater than they were in the preceding fiscal year are more complicated than the formula used when Part B appropriations are less than they were in the preceding year. A Part B appropriation equal to or greater than the previous year's appropriation is also the more common scenario, occurring in 36 of the 40 years between FY1977 and FY2017 (as displayed in *Figure 1*).[41] The calculations used in years when Part B funding increases or remains the same are outlined below.

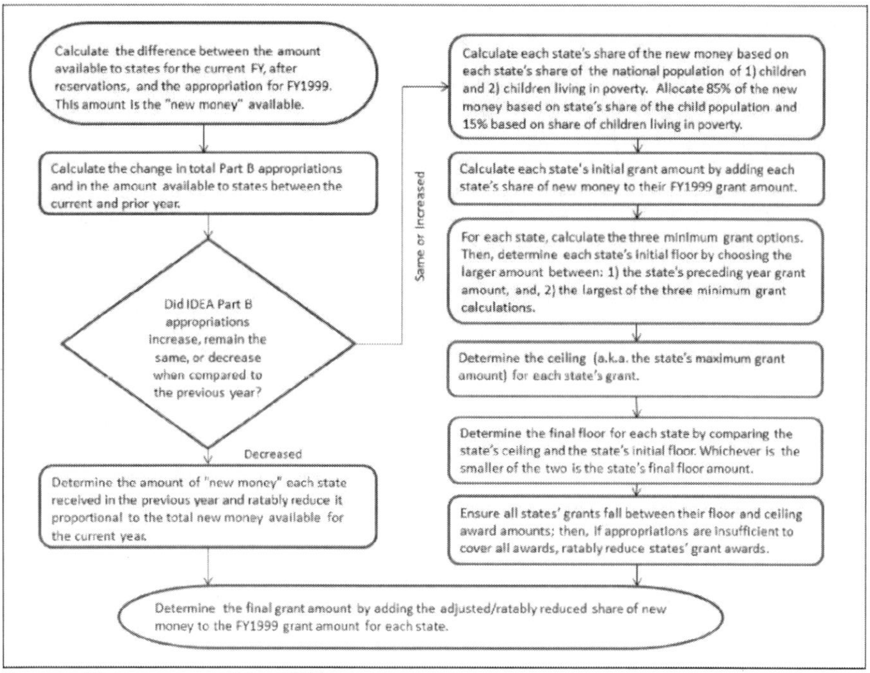

Source: Figure prepared by CRS.

Figure 2. Overview of the IDEA Part B Formula for Determining Grants to States.

---

[41] Funding for IDEA Part B grants to states was less than it had been the previous year in FY1996, FY2006, FY2011, and FY2013. Part B funding remained the same between FY1980 and FY1981 and FY2009 and FY2010. In all other years, Part B funding increased.

Basic IDEA State Grant Funding Calculation

As discussed previously, the base formula for state allocations was historically designed to target funds toward states with higher proportions of children with disabilities. After concerns arose that an IDEA formula based on the number of children found eligible for special education services in a state might incentivize special education placement and contribute to the disproportionate number of minority students receiving special education services, Congress changed the base formula during the reauthorization of the IDEA in 1997 to target funds toward states with larger total populations of children ages 3 through 21 years old, not specifically children with disabilities. In the current IDEA Part B formula, states with higher rates of children living in poverty are also targeted.

Currently, the basic formula for allocating Part B grants, in years when appropriations to states are equal to the prior year or have increased, remains the same as the one put in place during the 1997 reauthorization of the IDEA. Under this formula, 85% of any funds over the base-year appropriation (FY1999) are distributed based on the state's share of the United States' total population of children ages 3 through 21,[42] and the remaining 15% is distributed according to the state's share of children of the same age range living in poverty.

Each state's initial Part B grant is the sum of three factors: the state's FY1999 base-year grant, the state's share of new money based on population, and the state's share of new money based on poverty. The second two factors are calculated using the state's share of the national population of children ages 3 through 21 and the state's share of children living in poverty. Each state's share of the national child population is calculated by dividing a state's total population of children[43] by the national population of children ages 3 through 21; and each state's share of the national population of children in poverty is calculated by dividing the

[42] Currently 18 states, the District of Columbia, and Puerto Rico provide children a free appropriate public education until the age of 21, the remaining states stop providing FAPE to students at 18, 19, or 20 years of age. The population used in IDEA formula calculations is based on the age range served in each state. A list of the age ranges served in each state can be found in *Table A-1* in *Appendix A* of this chapter.

[43] See footnote 42.

state's population of children living in poverty by the U.S. population of children living in poverty.

$$State\ Share_{Pop} = \frac{Child\ Pop_{State}}{Child\ Pop_{US}}$$

$$State\ Share_{Pov} = \frac{Child\ Pov_{State}}{Child\ Pov_{US}}$$

To calculate fully the initial Part B grant for an individual state, one first has to determine the state's grant based on the state's population of children ages 3 through 21 and the state's grant based on their share of children ages 3 through 21 living in poverty. State grants based on population (*State* $Grant_{pop}$) are calculated by allocating 85% of the "new money" (i.e., funds over the FY1999 base-year appropriation) based on the state's share of the U.S. child population, and state grants based on poverty (*State* $Grant_{pov}$) are calculated by allocating 15% of the new Part B money based on the state's share of the U.S. child population living in poverty.

$$State\ Grant_{Pop} = 85\%\ of\ New\ Money \times State\ Share_{Pop}$$

$$State\ Grant_{Pov} = 15\%\ of\ New\ Money \times State\ Share_{Pov}$$

Each state's initial Part B grant is the sum of the state's FY1999 base-year grant, their initial state grant based on population, and their initial state grant based on poverty.

$$Basic\ State\ Grant = Grant_{FY1999} + State\ Grant_{Pop} + State\ Grant_{Pov}$$

Once each state's initial or "basic" grant has been calculated it may be adjusted based on each state's minimum and maximum grant levels, which also must be calculated. If the initial grant a state would receive based on the basic IDEA funding formula would fall outside the range determined by the minimum and maximum grant calculations, the state's IDEA grant is set to its floor or ceiling grant allocation as appropriate.

Allocation Floor

Part B describes four amounts used to determine a state's minimum grant amount or allocation floor. First, determine each of these four amounts; then set the largest of them as the state's allocation floor.

The first amount is the state's preceding-year allocation, commonly known as the "hold harmless" amount.[44] The other three amounts are calculated using three formulas for minimum grant amounts outlined in the IDEA:

1. Calculate the first state minimum grant award amount by adding the FY1999 award level for a state and 1⁄3% (i.e., 0.0033) of the amount by which the current year's (CY) appropriation exceeds the amount appropriated for Part B in FY1999:

$$\text{Minimum}_1 = \text{Grant}_{FY1999} + ((\text{Appropriation}_{CY} - \text{Appropriation}_{FY1999}) \times 0.0033)$$

   This calculation only results in the highest minimum grant award amount for states with small populations, and therefore is sometimes referred to as the "small state minimum."

2. Calculate the second state minimum grant award amount by adding the state's prior-year (PY) award level, and that prior-year amount multiplied by any percentage increase in appropriations for Part B in excess of 1.5% above the preceding fiscal year's appropriation:

$$\text{Minimum}_2 = \text{Grant}_{PY} + \left(\text{Grant}_{PY} \times \left(\left(\frac{\text{ApropIncrease}_{CY-PY}}{\text{Approp}_{PY}}\right) - 0.015\right)\right)$$

   This calculation results in the greatest minimum allocation for states in years when there is a large (e.g., >15%) increase in the amount appropriated for Part B.

---

[44] The hold harmless provision states that "no State's allocation shall be less than its allocation under this section for the preceding fiscal year." 20 U.S.C. §1411(d)(3)(B)(i); P.L. 108-446 §611(d)(3)(B)(i).

3. The third state minimum grant award is calculated by adding a state's prior-year award and that prior-year amount multiplied by 90% of the percentage increase in the amount appropriated for Part B from the preceding fiscal year.[45]

$$\text{Minimum}_3 = \text{Grant}_{PY} + \left(\text{Grant}_{PY} \times 0.9\left(\frac{\text{ApropIncrease}_{CY-PY}}{\text{Approp}_{PY}}\right)\right)$$

This calculation is used for most states in years when the increase in the Part B appropriation is less than 15% above the previous fiscal year. In practical terms, this third minimum state grant will always result in a grant amount equal to or greater than a state's preceding-year allocation.

The state's preceding-year allocation is compared to the results of three state award minimum calculations. The largest of these four quantities is then set as that state's allocation floor.

Allocation Ceiling

There is one calculation to determine each state's maximum award or ceiling (i.e., the amount the state's allocation may not exceed). The maximum award is calculated as the sum of the amount the state received the preceding fiscal year and that prior-year amount multiplied by the sum of 1.5% and the percentage increase in the amount appropriated from the preceding fiscal year.[46]

$$\text{Maximum Award} = \text{Grant}_{PY} + \left(\text{Grant}_{PY} \times \left(\left(\frac{\text{ApropIncrease}_{CY-PY}}{\text{Approp}_{PY}}\right) + 0.015\right)\right)$$

The maximum grant calculation is a unique component of the Part B formula. Most education funding formulas contain only minimum award levels or funding floors, but do not set a limit on the maximum funding a

45 20 U.S.C. §1411(d)(3)(B)(ii); P.L. 108-446 §611(d)(3)(B)(ii).
46 20 U.S.C. §1411(d)(3)(B)(iii), P.L. 108-446 §611(d)(3)(B)(iii).

state may receive. The maximum grant level allows for the possibility that some funds would be unallocated in years in which IDEA funding rises enough that every state can receive its maximum grant. In some cases, the calculated maximum award for a state is less than the calculated minimum for that state. When this happens, the state's final floor is set equal to its ceiling, and the state receives the lesser of the two amounts—the maximum award.

When Part B grants to the 50 states, the District of Columbia, and Puerto Rico for FY2015 (shown in *Table 2*) are examined, the majority of states (44 out of 52; 85%) received their minimum award amount. Only two of those states (Alaska and Montana) received the "small state minimum" allocation. In other words, the first of the three state-grant-award-minimum calculations (shown above) was used to determine minimum and final grant allocations for only two states. The other 42 states receiving their minimum award amount received the allocation derived from the third minimum state grant calculation.[47] As mentioned previously, the third minimum grant calculation is used for most states in years when the Part B appropriation is less than 15% greater than the previous fiscal year's appropriation. One state (Arizona) received a Part B grant allocation between its minimum and maximum grant. The remaining seven states received their maximum allocations.[48]

As stated previously, a state's maximum award is the amount the state's allocation *may not exceed*, as opposed to the maximum amount it *can receive*. And, when determining a state's final floor, the lesser amount between the minimum and maximum grant for the state is the amount awarded. Therefore, when a state's maximum grant is lower than the state's highest calculated minimum grant, the maximum grant amount is allocated. This can be seen in the cases of the states awarded their maximum allocations in *Table 2*.

---

[47] The second formula is used in years when IDEA's appropriation increases more than 15%. Because Part B's appropriation increased 3.6% in this example, the third formula was the appropriate minimum allocation formula for all states not using the small state minimum formula.

[48] The seven states that received their maximum allocation were Delaware, the District of Columbia, Nevada, North Dakota, South Dakota, Vermont, and Wyoming.

Table 2. State Minimum, Maximum, and Final Grant Allocations for IDEA Part B, FY2018

State	Minimum Grant	Maximum Grant	Final Grant	Calculation
Alabama	$190,495,767	$193,723,104	$190,495,767	3rd Minimum
Alaska[a]	$38,804,517	$39,324,225	$38,804,517	1st Minimum
Arizona	$207,805,274	$211,325,866	$211,325,866	Maximum
Arkansas	$117,332,895	$119,320,723	$117,332,895	3rd Minimum
California	$1,281,755,429	$1,303,470,649	$1,281,755,429	3rd Minimum
Colorado[b]	$167,004,880	$169,834,241	$167,500,962	3rd Minimum*
Connecticut	$139,540,151	$141,904,209	$139,540,151	3rd Minimum
Delaware[a]	$37,781,829	$38,262,766	$37,781,829	1st Minimum
District of Columbia	$32,200,957	$19,667,309	$19,667,309	Maximum
Florida	$674,522,024	$685,949,629	$674,522,024	3rd Minimum
Georgia	$355,374,234	$361,394,907	$361,394,907	Maximum
Hawaii	$41,721,163	$42,427,994	$41,721,163	3rd Minimum
Idaho[b]	$58,917,758	$59,915,930	$59,266,522	3rd Minimum*
Illinois	$530,733,888	$539,725,466	$530,733,888	3rd Minimum
Indiana	$271,331,688	$275,928,530	$271,331,688	3rd Minimum
Iowa	$128,160,856	$130,332,129	$128,160,856	3rd Minimum
Kansas	$111,927,946	$113,824,205	$111,927,946	3rd Minimum
Kentucky	$165,732,139	$168,539,936	$165,732,139	3rd Minimum
Louisiana	$197,709,365	$201,058,914	$197,709,365	3rd Minimum
Maine	$57,442,824	$58,416,007	$57,442,824	3rd Minimum
Maryland	$209,867,861	$213,423,396	$209,867,861	3rd Minimum
Massachusetts	$297,998,648	$303,047,276	$297,998,648	3rd Minimum
Michigan	$418,811,813	$425,907,231	$418,811,813	3rd Minimum
Minnesota	$198,984,329	$202,355,478	$198,984,329	3rd Minimum
Mississippi	$125,613,268	$127,741,380	$125,613,268	3rd Minimum
Missouri	$238,429,634	$242,469,057	$238,429,634	3rd Minimum
Montanaa	$39,554,764	$40,102,915	$39,554,764	1st Minimum
Nebraska	$78,386,951	$79,714,966	$78,386,951	3rd Minimum
Nevada	$78,948,562	$80,286,091	$80,286,091	Maximum
New Hampshire	$49,813,585	$50,657,516	$49,813,585	3rd Minimum
New Jersey	$379,450,638	$385,879,208	$379,450,638	3rd Minimum
New Mexico	$95,616,693	$97,236,610	$95,616,693	3rd Minimum
New York	$796,284,914	$809,775,399	$796,284,914	3rd Minimum
North Carolina	$353,310,198	$359,295,903	$353,310,198	3rd Minimum
North Dakota	$35,671,456	$31,761,185	$31,761,185	Maximum
Ohio	$457,817,083	$465,573,320	$457,817,083	3rd Minimum
Oklahoma	$155,678,097	$158,315,561	$155,678,097	3rd Minimum
Oregon	$135,038,537	$137,326,331	$135,038,537	3rd Minimum
Pennsylvania	$446,896,819	$454,468,048	$446,896,819	3rd Minimum
Rhode Island	$45,906,938	$46,684,683	$45,906,938	3rd Minimum

State	Minimum Grant	Maximum Grant	Final Grant	Calculation
South Carolina	$185,645,704	$188,790,873	$185,645,704	3rd Minimum
South Dakota[a]	$37,414,658	$37,835,833	$37,414,658	1st Minimum
Tennessee	$249,311,747	$253,535,532	$249,311,747	3rd Minimum
Texas[b]	$1,057,502,718	$1,075,418,698	$1,068,318,577	3rd Minimum*
Utah	$118,743,627	$120,755,355	$120,755,355	Maximum
Vermont	$35,345,081	$30,623,846	$30,623,846	Maximum
Virginia	$298,099,751	$303,150,091	$298,099,751	3rd Minimum
Washington	$231,413,434	$235,333,990	$231,413,434	3rd Minimum
West Virginia	$79,725,309	$81,075,998	$79,725,309	3rd Minimum
Wisconsin	$218,219,467	$221,916,493	$218,219,467	3rd Minimum
Wyoming	$35,776,560	$32,127,451	$32,127,451	Maximum
Puerto Rico	$125,705,692	$127,835,370	$127,835,370	Maximum

Source: Prepared by CRS based on unpublished data provided by the U.S. Department of Education (ED), Budget Service.

[a] Four states—Alaska, Delaware, Montana, and South Dakota—received their "small state minimum" grant in FY2018.

[b] Three states—Colorado, Idaho, and Texas—received a modified version of their third minimum.

Final Part B State Grant Funding Calculation

Once each state's floor and ceiling amounts are calculated, those amounts are compared to the initial grant amount calculated based upon population and poverty data. Each state's grant amount must be adjusted to fit within the range of its floor and ceiling grant levels. States' initial grant amounts that fall outside this range are either brought up to equal their floors or brought down to equal their ceilings.

If sufficient funds are not available to fully cover the calculated grant levels, ratable reduction is used to arrive at allocations across the states. During the ratable reduction process, no state's grant amount may be reduced below its prior-year allocation or its hold harmless level.[49] Final state grant amounts are calculated by adding each state's adjusted and ratably reduced new money grant and the state's FY1999 base-year grant.

Decreased Federal Funding IDEA Part B Funding

If the amount appropriated for Part B grants is below the amount appropriated for the preceding fiscal year but above the amount appropriated

[49] 20 U.S.C. §1411(d)(3)(C), P.L. 108-446 §611(d)(3)(C).

in FY1999, a single calculation is used. Each state is allocated the sum of its FY1999 base-year grant and an amount of the current fiscal year's Part B new money proportional to the share of new money the state received the prior fiscal year.[50]

First, calculate the amount of new money provided to each state the previous year:

$$New\ Money_{State\_PY} = Grant_{PY} - Grant_{FY1999}$$

After totaling the new money available to all states in the previous year, calculate each state's ratably reduced funding amount for the current year:

$$State\ Grant_{CY} = \frac{New\ Money_{State\_PY}}{New\ Money_{US\_PY}} \times New\ Money_{CY}$$

Determine the final grant amount for each state by adding the state's ratably reduced new money grant amount to the state's FY1999 grant amount.

$$Final\ State\ Grant = State\ Grant_{CY} + StateGrant_{FY1999}$$

If Congress provided the Part B program an annual appropriation less than or equal to the amount it provided in FY1999,[51] a single, simpler calculation would be used.[52] The amount each state received in FY1999 would be ratably reduced based on the amount of the reduction in overall funding for the program. This calculation has not been used to date. In FY2018, the IDEA grants-to-states program was appropriated $12.3 billion, $8 billion more than it received in FY1999, suggesting it may be unlikely IDEA funding will drop below FY1999 levels in the future.

[50] 34 C.F.R. §300.701(d)(1).
[51] The FY1999 IDEA Part B appropriation was $4,301,000,000.
[52] 20 U.S.C. §1411(d)(4)(A); P.L. 108-446 §611(d)(4)(A).

Grants to LEAs

States may reserve a portion of their federal IDEA funding for statewide activities,[53] but they are required to distribute the majority of their IDEA allocation to local educational agencies (LEAs) and public charter schools that operate as LEAs. In order for states to allocate IDEA funds to individual LEAs they must use a formula similar to the one used to divide IDEA funds among states, except that the sources of population and poverty data vary from state to state. First, the states are required to award each LEA an amount based on its FY1999 base-year allocation. Then states distribute the remaining allocation according to the share of the population of children in both public and private schools in the LEA (85%) and the LEA's share of children living in poverty (15%). If a state educational agency determines that an LEA is providing a free appropriate public education to all children with disabilities in the LEA using only state and local funds, the SEA may reallocate any unneeded federal IDEA Part B funds to other LEAs in the state that are not adequately providing FAPE to all the children with disabilities they serve.[54]

Grants for IDEA Early Childhood Programs

Preschool Grants Program (Part B, Section 619)

Section 619 of IDEA Part B authorizes grants to states for preschool programs serving children with disabilities ages three to five. Because Part B grants to states are used to serve children with disabilities as young as three years of age (as well as school-aged children), Section 619 is not so

---

[53] State activities include state administration, technical assistance, personnel preparation, professional development and training, supporting or improving the use of technology in the classroom by children with disabilities (including assistive technology devices) to enhance learning and maximize accessibility to the general education curriculum, developing and implementing transition programs, or assisting LEAs in meeting personnel shortages. For the full list of state activities and the amount states may reserve for state activities, see 20 U.S.C. §1411(e), P.L. 108-446 §611(e).

[54] 20 U.S.C. §1411(f)(3), P.L. 108-446 §611(f)(3).

much a separate program as it is supplementary funding for services to preschool children with disabilities. In general, the provisions, requirements, and guarantees under the grants-to-states program that apply to school-age children with disabilities also apply to children in this age group.

Part B, Section 619 preschool grants follow the calculations previously discussed for determining Part B grants to states for children ages 3 through 21 years old, with the following adjustments:

- The reservation for administration and state-level activities that states may reserve from their Part B, Section 619 grant awards is greater than the amount states may reserve from their larger Part B, Section 611 grants (25% vs. 5%).
- Where the FY1999 grant is used in a calculation to determine "Part B Grants to States," it is replaced by the FY1997 grant in Part B, Section 619 calculations.[55]

Infants and Families Program (IDEA Part C)

The calculations used to determine the IDEA Part C infants and families program grants are simpler than those used for either of the Part B grant programs. After the Secretary has reserved funds for payments to the outlying areas,[56] and for tribes, tribal organizations, and consortia of those groups for the provision of early intervention services on reservations,[57] the

---

[55] The funding formula adopted through the 1997 IDEA amendments for the grants-to-states program took effect the year the federal appropriation for the grants-to-states program first exceeded $4.9 billion. Because the IDEA grants-to-states program appropriation first exceeded $4.9 billion in FY2000, the base-year amount states were guaranteed for their Part B, Section 611 grant was their FY1999 funding level. However, Part B, Section 619 does not include a similar appropriation level that must be exceeded to establish a base-year amount; instead it uses the year the new funding formula was adopted (i.e., FY1997) as its base year in all calculations.

[56] 20 U.S.C. §1411(b)(1); P.L. 108-446 §616(b)(1). The outlying areas are defined in §602(22) as the "United States Virgin Islands, Guam, American Samoa, and the Commonwealth of the Northern Mariana Islands." Part C §643(2) further states "The provisions of Public Law 95–134, permitting the consolidation of grants to the outlying areas, shall not apply to funds those areas receive under this part."

[57] Section 643(b)(1) reserves 1.25% of the Part C appropriation for the Department of the Interior for the "coordination of assistance in the provision of early intervention services by the States to infants and toddlers with disabilities and their families on reservations served by

Secretary allocates the remaining IDEA Part C amount among the 50 states, the District of Columbia, and Puerto Rico according to the ratio of infants and toddlers in each state to the number of infants and toddlers in all states. The minimum allotment for each state is either $500,000 or one-half of 1% of the total Part C funds allotted to the states, whichever is greater.[58] If the appropriation for Part C is funded at a level insufficient to pay the full amounts that all states are eligible to receive in a given year, the Secretary must ratably reduce the states' payments, meaning the reduction will be proportionately reflected in the allotment for each state, including states initially receiving the minimum Part C grant amount.[59]

IDEA FUNDING ISSUES

Full Funding

The amount required to provide the maximum amount for each state's grant is commonly referred to as "full funding" of the IDEA. When Congress enacted the predecessor legislation to the IDEA in 1975, they strove to ensure that (1) states would provide every eligible child FAPE in the least restrictive environment, and (2) states would not take on an untenable financial burden by agreeing to provide special education and related services.

At the time, the available estimate of the cost of educating children with disabilities was, on average, twice the cost of educating other children. A determination was made that the federal government would pay some of this

---

elementary schools and secondary schools for Indian children operated or funded by the Department of the Interior."

[58] $500,000 is one half of 1% of $100 million. Part C of the IDEA has been appropriated more than $100,000,000 every year since FY1991. Therefore, in practice, the minimum Part C allotment for each state is one half of 1% of the IDEA Part C appropriation available to be allocated to states; in recent years, this has been over $2,000,000.

[59] If additional funds become available for making payments for a fiscal year in which payments to states were ratably reduced, the allotments that were reduced must be increased on the same basis the allotments were reduced. §643(c)(3).

additional or "excess" cost. The metric for determining this excess cost was the national average per-pupil expenditure (APPE). Congress's final determination was that the federal government would pay up to 40% of the excess cost of providing special education and related services, and 40% of the national APPE adjusted by the number of children with disabilities a state served came to be known as the "full funding" amount of IDEA Part B grants to states.

IDEA funding has fallen short of the full funding amount each year from the formula's enactment through FY2018. For example, in FY2018 the amount appropriated for Part B accounted for approximately 15% of the national APPE, less than half of the 40% full funding level. In FY2009, Part B appropriations approached closer to the full funding amount than they had before or have since, when, with the addition of federal stimulus dollars, IDEA funding rose to almost 35% of the APPE.

Prior to the enactment of P.L. 108-446 in 2004, the maximum amount a state could receive under the Part B grants-to-states program was based on 40% of the national APPE multiplied by the number of children with disabilities the state serves.[60] P.L. 108-446 changed the method of calculating the maximum amount of states' grants.

A state's maximum grant amount for purposes of calculating "full funding" differs from the maximum grant level calculation performed in years when the IDEA Part B appropriation has increased, as described earlier in this chapter. The maximum grant level calculation described earlier is used in years when the most common funding scenario occurs—IDEA Part B appropriations increase but remain below the full funding level. In contrast, the maximum amount of each state's grant for the purposes of full funding would only be calculated in a year when IDEA Part B was fully funded. A state may never receive more than its full funding maximum grant amount, even if Congress were to appropriate more than the amount necessary to fully fund all state grant awards.

P.L. 108-446 set a new calculation to determine the maximum amount of state grants under full-funding. Beginning in FY2007 and used for all

[60] P.L. 105-17 §611(a)(2).

subsequent fiscal years, the maximum amount of state grants for the purposes of full funding has been calculated as 40% of APPE multiplied by the number of children with disabilities the state served in school year 2004-2005, and then adjusted by the annual rates of change in the state's population in the age range comparable to ages for which the state provides FAPE for children with disabilities[61] (85% of the adjustment) and in the state's population of children living in poverty in the same age range (15% of the adjustment).[62] That is, a state's maximum grant amount or full funding level under the Part B grant-to-states program is 40% of APPE multiplied by the number of children with disabilities served and adjusted for each state's annual changes in child population and poverty rate.[63]

Prior to the enactment of P.L. 108-446, the IDEA authorized "such sums as may be necessary" for the Part B grants-to-states program. In response to debate over how and when to reach full funding for the IDEA, P.L. 108-446 (§611(i)) amended the act to include several years of specific authorization levels, which culminated in an amount estimated to provide each state with its maximum grant amount in FY2011. The Part B grants-to-states program was not appropriated the amounts authorized by P.L. 108-446 and did not obtain full funding in FY2011.

Maintenance of Effort (MOE)

The IDEA was intended to help states and LEAs increase overall educational spending, rather than substituting federal funds for education

[61] For most states this age range is 3 to 20 or 3 to 21.

[62] For example, if a state's relevant population for school year 2007-2008 rose by 3% above its 2004-2005 population and its number of children living in poverty rose by 2% above the 2004-2005 number, then its 2007-2008 maximum grant would be the appropriate APPE for that year multiplied by the 2004-2005 number of children with disabilities served increased by 2.85% (85% of 3% plus 15% of 2% = 2.55% + 0.3% = 2.85%).

[63] See Section 611(a)(2)(B) of IDEA. Under P.L. 108-446, the calculation of maximum state grants changed in FY2007. For more information, congressional clients may request archived CRS Report RL32716, *Individuals with Disabilities Education Act (IDEA): Analysis of Changes Made by* P.L. 108-446, for a discussion of this change.

spending at the state and local levels. The grants to states made under Part B may only be used to pay for the excess costs of providing special education and related services to students with disabilities[64] and may not replace state or local funding. To these ends, the IDEA contains supplement, not supplant (SNS) and maintenance of effort (MOE) requirements. IDEA's SNS requirements prohibit a state or LEA from using IDEA grants to provide services, purchase equipment, etc., that state, local, or other federal funds currently provide or purchase or, in the absence of the IDEA funds, would have provided or purchased. The IDEA MOE provisions require that a state or an LEA not reduce their support for special education and related services below the level of support provided the previous fiscal year.[65]

In general, a state may not reduce the amount of state financial *support* for special education and related services for children with disabilities below the amount of that support for the preceding fiscal year.[66] In any fiscal year in which a state does not meet this MOE requirement, the Secretary of Education is required to reduce the state's subsequent year grant by the same amount by which the state fails to meet the requirement.[67] States support special education in different ways and through a variety of agencies;[68] however, for each state to meet the MOE provision of the IDEA, it must provide support for special education at no lower than the same aggregate level each year as it did in the preceding fiscal year. As long as a state maintains its level of financial support for special education from one year

---

[64] For more information on Part B of the IDEA see CRS Report R41833, The Individuals with Disabilities Education Act (IDEA), Part B: Key Statutory and Regulatory Provisions.

[65] Exceptions to the basic requirements of MOE are discussed in "Reduction of MOE Requirements: States" and "Reduction in MOE: LEAs," in this chapter.

[66] 20 U.S.C. §1412(a)(18)(A); P.L. 108-446 §612(a)(18)(A).

[67] 20 U.S.C. §1412(a)(18)(B); P.L. 108-446 §612(a)(18)(B).

[68] For example, in Office of Special Education Programs (OSEP) Memorandum 10-5, ED explains that while SEAs provide most of the special education and related services and therefore supervise the majority of the federal IDEA funds appropriated to the state, other state agencies such as the State Vocational Rehabilitation Agency or the State Department of Health may provide children with disabilities services pursuant to their IEPs, and their contributions to providing IEP services would be included in the "State financial support for special education and related services for children with disabilities," that must be maintained to meet the MOE requirement. Letter from Alexa Posny, Acting Director of OSEP, U.S. Department of Education, to Chief State School Officers, State Directors of Special Education, December 2, 2009, http://www2.ed.gov/policy/speced/guid/idea/ letters/2009-4/index.html.

to the next, the level of financial support for special education and related services in a state may be maintained by a combination of state agencies, including, but not necessarily limited to, the state educational agency (SEA).

The MOE provision for LEAs is similar to the MOE provision for states. However, the LEA may not "reduce the level of expenditures for the education of children with disabilities made by the local educational agency from local funds below the level of those expenditures for the preceding fiscal year."[69] At the local level, the individual LEAs, and no other local agencies, are responsible for maintaining their levels of IDEA expenditures from one fiscal year to the next. Stated another way, states and LEAs are both responsible for maintaining effort, however, states may count contributions to SEAs and other state agencies to meet this requirement, while LEAs must maintain their level of expenditures on special education themselves—they may not consider funds provided to other agencies in order to maintain their level of effort. The key difference between the state and LEA MOE requirements pertains to whether a single agency or multiple agencies bear the responsibility for maintaining financial effort.

As noted above, if a state or LEA fails to meet the MOE requirement in any fiscal year, its funding allocation will be reduced during the next fiscal year in the amount by which it failed to meet the requirement.[70] However, for both states and LEAs there are permissible reasons for reductions in MOE requirements; these reasons are discussed next.

Reduction of MOE Requirements: States

In certain rare instances a state may be granted a one-year waiver of the MOE requirement. The Secretary may grant a waiver, for one fiscal year at a time, in the case of "exceptional or uncontrollable circumstances" such as a natural disaster or a "precipitous and unforeseen decline in the financial resources of the state."[71] In addition, waivers can be granted if the state can

---

[69] 20 U.S.C. §1413(a)(2)(A)(iii); P.L. 108-446 §613(a)(2)(A)(iii).
[70] States: 20 U.S.C. §1412(a)(18)(B); LEAs: 20 U.S.C. §1413(d).
[71] This type of waiver has been granted in the past. See http://www2.ed.gov/policy/speced/guid/idea/monitor/smfspartb-waivers.html for links to state waiver applications and ED's letters of response. 20 U.S.C. §1412(a)(18)(C)(i), P.L. 108-446 §612(a)(18)(C)(i).

provide "clear and convincing evidence" that FAPE is available for all children with disabilities in the state.[72] Proving that FAPE is available to every eligible child with a disability in the state is a high standard and, since the MOE provisions were first included in the IDEA in 1997, this type of waiver has never been granted.

If a state does not meet its MOE requirement for any given year, including any year for which the state was granted a waiver, the state financial support required in future years is not reduced. That is, the state must provide the amount that would have been required in the absence of failing to meet MOE in the previous year.[73] A waiver will reduce a state's financial support requirement for the year it is granted but not for subsequent years. A penalty may be imposed on a state for any fiscal year after the fiscal year the state reduces its special education funding.

Reduction of MOE Requirements: LEAs

LEAs vary in size, from large urban districts like New York City Public Schools and Los Angeles Unified School District to individual charter schools that operate as their own LEAs. Small LEAs, which lack the benefits economies of scale provide to large school districts, may find their special education budgets varying considerably from one year to the next due to changes in their staffing or student population. The IDEA potentially allows any LEA to reduce educational expenditures below the level of the preceding fiscal year if the reduction is attributable to

- the voluntary departure (e.g., by retirement) or departure for just cause of special education personnel;
- a decrease in enrollment of students with disabilities;
- the termination of an obligation to provide an individual child with a disability an exceptionally costly program, either because the child moved out of the LEA's jurisdiction, graduated, aged out of special education services, or no longer needs the program;

---

[72] 20 U.S.C. §1412(a)(18)(C)(ii); P.L. 108-446 §612(a)(18)(C)(ii).
[73] 20 U.S.C. §1412(a)(18)(D); P.L. 108-446 §612(a)(18)(D).

- the termination of costly expenditures for long-term purchases such as the acquisition of equipment or construction of school facilities;
- the assumption of cost by the high-cost fund/high-risk pool operated by the SEA under the IDEA provisions for high-cost funds; or[74]
- an increase in the allocation of IDEA funds from the previous year that allows an LEA to employ the "50%" rule.[75]

ED has clarified in its policy letters that an LEA's reduction in MOE should only be for one of the reasons on this list.[76] When the Minnesota Department of Education wanted to know if an LEA's increased efficiency at providing services and its subsequent cost savings could justify a reduction in MOE, providing the example of an LEA that consolidated bus routes, ED's response was two-fold. Increased efficiency alone is not a suitable reason to allow an LEA to reduce its MOE according to ED. However, if the LEA could explain how the increased efficiency was attributable to one of the circumstances outlined in the statute (listed as the six bullet points above), it could potentially justify the reduction in spending.

High Cost Pools/Risk Pools

As previously mentioned, when Congress enacted the predecessor legislation to IDEA in 1975,[77] the assumption was that education for children

[74] 34 C.F.R. §300.204.

[75] The 50% rule states "for any fiscal year for which the allocation received by a local educational agency under section 611(f) [of the IDEA] exceeds the amount the local educational agency received for the previous fiscal year, the local educational agency may reduce the level of expenditures...by not more than 50 percent of the amount of such excess." In addition, it requires the LEA to "use an amount of local funds equal to the reduction in expenditures...to carry out activities authorized under the Elementary and Secondary Education Act of 1965." 20 U.S.C. §1413(a)(2)(C) P.L. 108- 446 §613(a)(2)(C); 34 C.F.R. §300.205.

[76] Letter from Melody Musgrove, OSEP Director, to Carol Hokenson, Manager, Minnesota Department of Education, January 30, 2013, http://www2.ed.gov/policy/speced/guid/idea/index.html.

[77] Education for All Handicapped Children Act, P.L. 94-142.

with disabilities was, on average, twice as costly as education for other children. While on average it is possible that this estimate was accurate, it did not account for the exceptional expenses of providing special education and related services to high-need/high-cost children with disabilities. The APPE for children with high-cost special needs can range from 3 to over 13 times more than the APPE for general education students.[78]

To help LEAs with the extraordinary costs of paying for the most expensive special education services, many states set up risk pools or high cost funds that LEAs may apply to for extra funding when they are required to provide special education services that meet state-determined criteria for "high need." The definition of a high-need child with a disability varies from state to state. Some states set a specific dollar amount above which a child's services are considered high cost/high need. Other states define a high-need child with a disability as a child for whom the LEA's expenditures are a certain number of times higher than the APPE for a general education student.

How states choose to provide additional funding to LEAs with high-need children with disabilities also varies. The state may choose to pay for a percentage of the additional costs with or without a spending cap. For example, a state could decide it will pay 50% of all expenses over $25,000 up to $100,000, or 75% of all expenses over $50,000 with no upper limit. A state may also base the amount given for each child on the total number of requests for funding from the risk pool received from all LEAs in the state in a given year. In such a scenario, funding may be distributed to LEAs on a prorated basis depending on the total number of requests the state received.

Amendments adopted in the 2004 reauthorization of the IDEA allow states to use 10% of their Part B funds reserved for state-level activities to

[78] The Special Education Expenditure Project defined the group of students who fell into the top 5% of the expenditure distribution in their study as the "high-expenditure" group. Jay Chambers, Yael Kidron, Angeline Spain, Characteristics of High-Expenditure Students with Disabilities, 1999-2000, Special Education Expenditure Project – CSEF, May 2004, retrieved from http://www.csef-air.org/publications/seep/national/Rpt8.pdf.

establish and make disbursements from a high-cost fund to LEAs.[79] Though this was the first inclusion of risk pools or high-cost funds in the IDEA, many states used risk pools prior to 2004. States that had risk pool systems in place could use authorized Part B funds to support their existing risk pools as long as their systems met federal requirements. Any state that wants to use Part B funds to support a local risk pool needs to follow IDEA provisions for risk pools, including the following requirements:

- The SEA, in consultation with the state's LEAs, will develop a definition of a "high-need child with a disability" that addresses the financial impact a high-need child has on the budget of the child's LEA; and defines a high-need child with a disability as a child for which the cost of providing special education and related services is greater than 3 times the APPE in the state.
- The SEA will develop a state plan establishing eligibility criteria for LEAs to participate in the risk pool system that takes into account the number and percentage of high-need children with disabilities served by an LEA.
- LEAs will only be allowed to use disbursements from risk pools to provide direct services outlined in the individualized education programs (IEPs) of high-cost children with disabilities.[80]

States may operate a risk pool or high-cost fund that does not meet these requirements provided no Part B funds are used to support their risk pool or high-cost fund.

---

[79] 20 U.S.C. §1412 (e)(3)(A).

[80] 20 U.S.C. §1412 (e)(3)(C to E). For more information on special education services and IEPs, see CRS Report R41833, *The Individuals with Disabilities Education Act (IDEA), Part B: Key Statutory and Regulatory Provisions*.

Appendix A. IDEA, Part B Age Ranges

Table A-1. IDEA, Part B Age Range Covered by State

State	Age Range (years)
Alabama	3–20
Alaska	3–21
Arizona	3–21
Arkansas	3–20
California	3–18
Colorado	3–20
Connecticut	3–20
Delaware	3–20
District of Columbia	3–21
Florida	3–21
Georgia	3–21
Hawaii	3–19
Idaho	3–20
Illinois	3–20
Indiana	3–21
Iowa	3–20
Kansas	3–20
Kentucky	3–20
Louisiana	3–21
Maine	3–19
Maryland	3–20
Massachusetts	3–21
Michigan	3–21
Minnesota	3–20
Mississippi	3–20
Missouri	3–20
Montana	3–18
Nebraska	3–20
Nevada	3–21
New Hampshire	3–20
New Jersey	3–20
New Mexico	3–21
New York	3–20
North Carolina	3–21
North Dakota	3–20
Ohio	3–21

State	Age Range (years)
Oklahoma	3–21
Oregon	3–20
Pennsylvania	3–20
Rhode Island	3–20
South Carolina	3–20
South Dakota	3–20
Tennessee	3–21
Texas	3–21
Utah	3–21
Vermont	3–21
Virginia	3–21
Washington	3–20
West Virginia	3–20
Wisconsin	3–20
Wyoming	3–20
Puerto Rico	3–21

Source: Information provided by U.S. Department of Education Budget Service in April 2018, as in effect in 2017.

The population used in IDEA formula calculations is based on the age range served in each state

APPENDIX B. COMMONLY USED ACRONYMS

APPE	Average Per Pupil Expenditure
APR	Annual Performance Report
CEIS	Coordinated Early Intervening Services
CY	Current Year
ED	U.S. Department of Education
ESEA	Elementary and Secondary Education Act
FAPE	Free Appropriate Public Education
FY	Fiscal Year
IDEA	The Individuals with Disabilities Education Act
IEP	Individualized Education Program
LEA	Local Educational Agency
MOE	Maintenance of Effort
PY	Prior Year

RTI	Response to Intervention
SEA	State Education Agency
SNS	Supplement, Not Supplant
SPP	State Performance Plan

In: Individuals with Disabilities
Editor: Aston Delgado
ISBN: 978-1-53615-030-8

Chapter 2

The Individuals with Disabilities Education Act (IDEA), Part B: Key Statutory and Regulatory Provisions (Updated)*

Kyrie E. Dragoo

Summary

The Individuals with Disabilities Education Act (IDEA) is a statute that authorizes grant programs that support special education services. Under the IDEA, a series of conditions are attached to the receipt of grant funds. These conditions aim to provide certain educational and procedural guarantees for students with disabilities and their families.

The grant programs authorized under the IDEA provide federal funding for special education and early intervention services for children with disabilities (birth to 21 years old) and require, as a condition for the receipt of such funds, the provision of a free appropriate public education (FAPE) (i.e., specially designed instruction provided at no cost to parents

* This is an edited, reformatted and augmented version of Congressional Research Service, Publication No. R41833, dated June 14, 2017.

that meets the needs of a child with a disability) and an accessible early intervention system (a statewide system to provide and coordinate early intervention services for infants and toddlers with disabilities and their families). The IDEA also outlines and requires the use of procedural safeguards pertaining to the identification, evaluation, and placement of students in special education services that are intended to protect the rights of parents and children with disabilities. These procedures include parental rights to resolve disputes through a mediation process, and present and resolve complaints through a due process complaint procedure and through state complaint procedures.

In the 2015-2016 school year, 6.8 million children ages 3 through 21 received educational services under Part B of the IDEA. To be covered under IDEA, a child with a disability must meet the categorical definition of disability in the act, and the child must require special education and related services as a result of the disability in order to benefit from public education. Once a child meets IDEA's eligibility criteria, FAPE is implemented through the Individualized Education Program (IEP), which is the plan for providing special education and related services by the local educational agency (LEA). The IEP is developed by an IEP team composed of school personnel and the child's parents or guardian. IDEA requires that children with disabilities be educated in the least restrictive environment. That is, to the maximum extent appropriate they are to be educated with children who are not disabled. In the fall of 2015, approximately 63% of all school-aged children with disabilities served by IDEA spent 80% or more of their time in a regular classroom.

To implement IDEA, states and other entities (i.e., the District of Columbia, Puerto Rico, the Bureau of Indian Education, the outlying areas, and the freely associated states) receive grants based on a statutory formula. In FY2017, $13.05 billion was appropriated for IDEA. Most of the federal funds received by states are passed on to LEAs based on a statutory formula. IDEA also contains state and local maintenance of effort (MOE) requirements and supplement, not supplant (SNS) requirements aimed at increasing overall educational spending, rather than substituting federal funds for education spending at the state and local levels.

Originally enacted in 1975, IDEA has been the subject of numerous reauthorizations to extend services and rights to children with disabilities. The most recent reauthorization of IDEA was P.L. 108-446, enacted in 2004. Funding for Part B, Assistance for Education of all Children with Disabilities, the largest and most often discussed part of the act, is permanently authorized. Funding for Part C, Infants and Toddlers with Disabilities, and Part D, National Activities, was authorized through FY2011. Funding for the programs continues to be authorized through annual appropriations.

INTRODUCTION

Background

The Individuals with Disabilities Education Act (IDEA) is the main federal statute governing special education for children from birth through age 21.[1] IDEA protects the rights of children with disabilities to a free appropriate public education (FAPE). It also supplements state and local funding to pay for some of the additional or excess costs of educating children with disabilities. IDEA is administered by the Office of Special Education Programs (OSEP) in the Office of Special Education and Rehabilitative Services (OSERS) in the Department of Education (ED). In the 2015-2016 school year (SY), 6.8 million children ages 3 through 21 received special education and related services under Part B of the IDEA.[2] In SY2015-2016, approximately 13.5% of all public school students ages 3 through 21 received services under the IDEA.[3]

IDEA was originally enacted in 1975 as the Education for All Handicapped Children Act, P.L. 94- 142.[4] At that time, Congress found that more than half of all children with disabilities were not receiving appropriate educational services and that 1 million children with disabilities were excluded entirely from the public school system. Further, Congress found that many of the children participating in regular school programs were prevented from having a successful educational experience because their

[1] 20 U.S.C. §1400 et seq.

[2] U.S. Department of Education, EDFacts Data Warehouse (EDW): "IDEA Part B Child Count and Educational Environments Collection," 2015-2016, http://www2.ed.gov/programs/osepidea/618-data/static-tables/index.html.

[3] CRS calculation based on U.S. Department of Education data in footnote 2 and National Center for Education Statistics, *Digest of Education Statistics*, Enrollment in public elementary and secondary schools, by level and grade: Selected years, fall 1980 through fall 2026, Table 203.10., https://nces.ed.gov/programs/digest/d16/tables/ dt16_203.10.asp.

[4] The name was changed to the Individuals with Disabilities Education Act by P.L. 101-476. The public law also substituted the phrase "children with disabilities" for the phrase "handicapped children" throughout the act.

disabilities were undiagnosed.[5] In addition to the awareness of the difficulties faced by children with disabilities, there were three other factors that precipitated the enactment of P.L. 94-142: (1) judicial decisions that found constitutional requirements for the education of children with disabilities, (2) the inability of states and localities to fund education for children with disabilities, and (3) potential long-term benefits of educating children with disabilities.[6]

IDEA consists of four parts. Part A contains the general provisions, including the purposes of the act and definitions. Part B contains provisions relating to the education of school aged children (the grants-to-states program) and state grants program for preschool children with disabilities (Section 619). Part C authorizes state grants for programs serving infants and toddlers with disabilities, while Part D contains the requirements for various national activities designed to improve the education of children with disabilities. Table 1 shows the structure and funding of IDEA. Appendix A provides a more detailed summary of each of the four parts.

Since 1975, IDEA has been the subject of numerous reauthorizations to extend services and rights to children with disabilities. The most recent reauthorization was P.L. 108-446 in 2004.[7] Funding for Part B, Assistance for Education of all Children with Disabilities, is permanently authorized. Funding for Part C, Infants and Toddlers with Disabilities, and Part D, National Activities, was authorized through FY2011.[8] Funding for the programs continues to be authorized through annual appropriations.

---

[5] 20 U.S.C. §1401(b), P.L. 94-142 §601(b).

[6] For more information on each of the factors that contributed to the enactment of P.L. 94-142, see CRS Report 95-669, *The Individuals with Disabilities Education Act: Congressional Intent*, by Nancy Lee Jones.

[7] For a discussion of the 2004 amendments made by P.L. 108-446, see CRS Report RL32716, *Individuals with Disabilities Education Act (IDEA): Analysis of Changes Made by P.L. 108-446*, by Ann Lordeman and Nancy Lee Jones. For an overview of the IDEA regulations from the Department of Education, see CRS Report RL33649, *The Individuals with Disabilities Education Act (IDEA): Final Regulations for P.L. 108-446*, and CRS Report R40055, *The Individuals with Disabilities Education Act: Final Part B Regulations*.

[8] IDEA authorizes appropriations for Part C and Part D programs and activities through FY2010. These authorities were automatically extended for an additional fiscal year by the General Education Provisions Act (GEPA; 20 U.S.C.§1226a). Funding for the programs continues to be authorized through annual appropriations.

Table 1. Structure and Funding of IDEA (Funding in thousands of dollars)

IDEA Part	Description	FY2017 Funding	Percentage of Total IDEA Funding
Part A—General Provisions	Includes findings, purposes, and definitions	—	—
Part B—Assistance for Education of all Children with Disabilities	Contains provisions relating to the education of school aged children (the grants-to-states program) and state grants program for preschool children with disabilities (Section 619)	$12,371,086[a]	94.8%
Part C—Infants and Toddlers with Disabilities	Authorizes state grants for programs serving infants and toddlers with disabilities	$458,556	3.5%
Part D—National Activities to Improve Education of Children with Disabilities	Contains the requirements for various national activities	$222,133	1.7%
IDEA Total		$13,051,775	100%

Source: Table prepared by CRS. Funding amounts are from Department of Education budget tables for FY2017.

[a] Of this amount, $368.2 million, or 2.8% of the total IDEA FY2017 appropriation, was appropriated for the state grants program for preschool children with disabilities (Section 619).

Three of the main purposes of IDEA are

(A) to ensure that all children with disabilities have available to them a free appropriate public education that emphasizes special education and related services designed to meet their unique needs and prepare them for further education, employment, and independent living; (B) to ensure that the rights of children with disabilities and parents of such children are protected; and (C) to assist states, localities, educational service agencies, and Federal agencies to provide for the education of all children with disabilities;[9]

The focus of this chapter will be on how these purposes are to be achieved under Part B of the IDEA, hereinafter referred to as IDEA. The first purpose is addressed primarily in the section of this chapter titled "Services for Children with Disabilities." The second is addressed in the section on "Procedural Safeguards," and the third is addressed in the section on "Funding, Expenditure Requirements, and Compliance."

SERVICES FOR CHILDREN WITH DISABILITIES

Children with disabilities receive specially designed instruction and other services to meet their unique needs. This section addresses (1) criteria children must meet to receive services under IDEA, (2) how the children are identified and evaluated, and (3) the procedures for developing an individualized education plan to provide special education and related services.

Children with Disabilities

To be covered under IDEA, a child with a disability must meet two criteria. First, the child must be in one of several categories of disabilities, and second, the child must require special education and related services as a result of the disability in order to benefit from public education.[10] If a child meets the two criteria, he or she would be eligible to receive specially

---

[9] 20 U.S.C. §1400(d)(1), P.L. 108-446 §601(d)(1).

[10] 20 U.S.C §14001(3)(A), P.L. 108-446 §602(3)(A), and 34 C.F.R. §300.8. The statute at §602(3)(B) also permits the state and LEA to include as a child with a disability a child age three through nine, or any subset of that range, who is experiencing developmental delays~as defined by the state and as measured by appropriate diagnostic instruments and proceduresin physical, cognitive, communication, social, emotional, or adaptive development. The child must also require special education and related services because of the developmental delay.

designed instruction or special education in which the content or the delivery of the instruction is adapted to the needs of the child.

Categories of Disabilities
Autism
Deaf-blindness
Deafness
Emotional disturbance
Hearing impairment
Intellectual disability[11]
Multiple disabilities
Orthopedic impairment
Other health impairment
Specific learning disability
Speech or language impairment
Traumatic brain injury
Visual impairment

If a child has a disability, but does not require special education to benefit from public education, he or she would not be covered under IDEA. The child might be covered, however, under two other acts that address the rights of individuals with disabilities: Section 504 of the Rehabilitation Act[12] and the Americans with Disabilities Act (ADA).[13] These two acts provide broad nondiscrimination protection not limited to education and have identical functional definitions of disability (i.e., disabilities related to such functions as seeing, hearing, walking, thinking) rather than the categorical definition used in the IDEA. "Several of the most common disabilities of

---

[11] P.L. 111-256, commonly referred to as Rosa's Law, required references to "mental retardation" in IDEA and other federal laws to change to "intellectual disability."

[12] 29 U.S.C. §794. For more information on Section 504, see CRS Report RL34041, *Section 504 of the Rehabilitation Act of 1973: Prohibiting Discrimination Against Individuals with Disabilities in Programs or Activities Receiving Federal Assistance*, coordinated by Cynthia Brown.

[13] 42 U.S.C. §12101 et seq. For a more detailed discussion of the ADA, see CRS Report 98-921, *The Americans with Disabilities Act (ADA): Statutory Language and Recent Issues*, by Cynthia Brown.

students included under Section 504 and the ADA, but not always covered under IDEA, are attention deficit hyperactivity disorder (ADHD), diabetes, and asthma."[14]

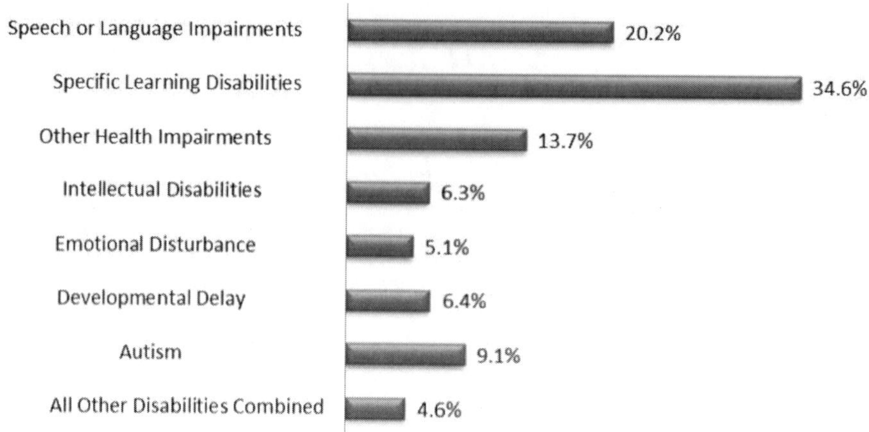

Source: U.S. Department of Education, EDFacts Data Warehouse (EDW): "IDEA Part B Child Count and Educational Environments Collection," 2015-2016, http://www2.ed.gov/programs/osepidea/618-data/index.html.

Notes: Percentages may not add to 100% because of rounding. Total number of students is 6.8 million.

"All other disabilities combined" include multiple disabilities, hearing impairments, orthopedic impairments, visual impairments, deaf-blindness, and traumatic brain injury.

"Developmental Delay" is a disability category that may be used at the discretion of the states for children ages 3 through 9 years old who are experiencing developmental delays in "one or more of the following areas: physical development; cognitive development; communication development; social or emotional development; or adaptive development." P.L. 108-446 §602(3)(B).

Figure 1. Disability Distribution for Students Ages 3 through 21 Receiving Special Education and Related Services under IDEA, Part B: Fall 2015.

---

[14] See citation to Rachel A. Holler and Perry A. Zirkel, "Section 504 and Public Schools: A National Survey Concerning 'Section 504-Only' Students," 92 NASSP Bulletin 19, 28 (March 2008) in CRS Report R40123, *Education of Individuals with Disabilities: The Individuals with Disabilities Education Act (IDEA), Section 504 of the Rehabilitation Act, and the Americans with Disabilities Act (ADA)*, by Nancy Lee Jones. For more information on differences among IDEA, Section 504, and the ADA, see this chapter.

Figure 1 shows the distribution of students with disabilities ages 3 through 21 receiving special education and related services in the fall of 2015. Approximately 35% of students with disabilities have specific learning disabilities (SLD).[15] Learning disabilities include such conditions as dyslexia, perceptual disabilities, and developmental aphasia.[16]

Free Appropriate Public Education (FAPE)

All children with disabilities receiving special education or related services under IDEA between the ages of 3 and 21, inclusive, residing in a state are entitled to FAPE.[17] The term "free appropriate public education" means:

> special education and related services that(A) have been provided at public expense, under public supervision and direction, and without charge; (B) meet the standards of the state educational agency; (C) include an appropriate preschool, elementary school, or secondary school education in the state involved; and (D) are provided in conformity with the individualized education program required under section 614(d) [Individualized Education Programs (IEP)].[18]

---

[15] A specific learning disability is defined as "a disorder in 1 or more of the basic psychological processes involved in understanding or in using language, spoken or written, which may manifest itself in the imperfect ability to listen, think, speak, read, write, spell, or do mathematical calculations." 20 U.S.C. §1401(30)(A), P.L. 108-446 §601(30)(A).

[16] 20 U.S.C. §1401(30)(B), P.L. 108-446 §601(30)(B). Specific learning disabilities do not include learning problems that are primarily the result of visual, hearing, or motor disabilities; of intellectual disability; of emotional disturbance; or of environmental, cultural, or economic disadvantage. 20 U.S.C §1401(30)(C), P.L. 108-446 §601(30)(C).

[17] The regulations at 34 C.F.R. §300.102 (2010) specify three exceptions to this requirement: (1) children ages 3, 4, 5, 18, 19, 20, or 21 in a state that does not provide a public education to children of those ages, (2) children ages 18 through 21 incarcerated in an adult correctional facility who were not identified as children with disabilities in their last educational placement; and (3) children with disabilities who have graduated from high school with a regular high school diploma.

[18] 20 U.S.C. §1401(9), P.L. 108-446 §601(9). For information on the legal aspects of FAPE, see CRS Report RL33444, *The Individuals with Disabilities Education Act (IDEA): Supreme Court Decisions*, by Nancy Lee Jones and Carol J. Toland; CRS Report R40521, *The Individuals with Disabilities Education Act (IDEA): Selected Judicial Developments Following the 2004 Reauthorization*, by Nancy Lee Jones; and CRS Report R40690, *The Individuals with*

FAPE must be made available to all children with disabilities who qualify for special education and related services, including children who have been suspended or expelled from school.[19]

Identification and Evaluation

Identifying and Evaluating a Child with a Disability

The first step in providing FAPE to children with disabilities is identifying them. Each state must have in effect policies and procedures to ensure that all children with disabilities residing in the state who are in need of special education and related services are identified, located, and evaluated. These policies and procedures are referred to in statute as "child find."[20] The children include those with disabilities who are

- homeless or wards of the state,
- attending private schools,
- suspected of having a disability, and
- highly mobile children, including migrant children.

A child who has been identified as having (or possibly having) a disability must be evaluated by the LEA before receiving special education and related services to determine whether a child is a child with a disability and to determine the educational needs of the child.[21] Either the parent or the LEA may request an initial evaluation.[22] In general, the LEA must obtain

---

Disabilities Education Act (IDEA): Statutory Provisions and Recent Legal Issues, coordinated by Cynthia Brown.

[19] 34 C.F.R. §300.101(a) (2010).

[20] 20 U.S.C §1412(a)(3), P.L. 108-446 §612(a)(3).

[21] 20 U.S.C. §1414(a), P.L. 108-446 §414(a). This subsection contains the requirements for evaluations, parental consent, and reevaluations.

[22] The LEA may refuse the parent's request for an initial evaluation if it does not suspect that the child has a disability. However, the public agency must provide written notice to the parents, consistent with 34 C.F.R. §300.503(b)(2010) and §615(c)(1) of the act, which explains, among other things, why the public agency refuses to conduct an initial evaluation and the information that was used as the basis to make that decision. The parent may challenge such a refusal by requesting a due process hearing. (71 Fed. Reg. 46636 (August 14, 2006)).

informed consent from the parent before conducting an initial evaluation.[23] Parental consent for an evaluation cannot be construed as consent for special education and related services.[24] The initial evaluation must take place within 60 days of receiving parental consent or within an alternative time frame established by the state.[25]

In conducting the initial evaluation, the LEA must

- use a variety of assessment tools and strategies to gather relevant functional, developmental, and academic information, including information provided by the parent;
- use multiple measures or assessments as the criteria for determining whether a child is a child with a disability or determining an appropriate educational program for the child; and
- use technically sound instruments that may assess the relative contribution of cognitive and behavioral factors, in addition to physical or developmental factors.[26]

In addition, assessments and other evaluation materials used to assess a child must be selected and administered so as not to be discriminatory on a racial or cultural basis. They must also be provided and administered in the language and form most likely to yield accurate information on what the child knows and can do academically, developmentally, and functionally.[27]

Upon completion of the evaluation, the determination of whether the child is a child with a disability is made and the educational needs of the

---

[23] The term "consent" is defined at 34 C.F.R. §300.9, and means, in part, that "the parent has been fully informed of all information relevant to the activity for which consent is sought, in his or her native language, or other mode of communication"; For more information on parental consent, see also 34 C.F.R. §300.300 (2010).

[24] In addition, at the time of the referral or parent request for evaluation, the LEA must provide the parent with the "Procedural Safeguards Notice," which is a comprehensive written explanation of IDEA's legal rights and protections for children with disabilities and their parents. See 20 U.S.C. §1415(d), P.L. 108-446 §615(d). For further information on procedural safeguards, see "Procedural Safeguards" in this chapter.

[25] 20 U.S.C §1414(a)(1), P.L. 108-446 §614 (a)(1).

[26] 20 U.S.C. §1414(b)(2), P.L. 108-446 §614 (b)(2).

[27] For all the provisions related to additional requirements, see 20 U.S.C. §1414(b)(3), P.L. 108-446 §614 (b)(3).

child are decided by a team of individuals that includes qualified professionals and the child's parent or guardian.[28] A copy of the evaluation report and the documentation of determination of eligibility must be provided to the parent.[29] In making a determination of eligibility, a child shall not be determined to be a child with a disability if the determinant factor is lack of appropriate instruction in reading, lack of instruction in math, or limited English proficiency.[30]

Reevaluations are required if the child's teacher or parent makes a request or if the LEA determines that the child's educational and service needs, academic achievement, or functional performance warrant a reevaluation. For example, a reevaluation might be warranted if the child's performance in school significantly improves, suggesting that he or she no longer requires special education and related services, or if the child is not making progress toward the goals in his or her IEP, indicating that changes are needed in the education or related services the LEA is providing. A reevaluation may not be done more than once a year unless the parent and LEA agree, and must be done at least once every three years unless the parent and the LEA agree that a reevaluation is not necessary.[31] In general, parental consent is required for reevaluations as well as for the initial evaluation.[32] In addition, the LEA cannot change the eligibility of a child until a reevaluation is done, unless the child graduates from high school with a regular diploma or reaches the age at which state law no longer provides for FAPE.[33]

Identifying and Evaluating a Child with a Specific Learning Disability (SLD)

As noted above, more than a third of children ages 3 through 21 receiving special education and related services under IDEA have SLDs. It

---

[28] 20 U.S.C. §1414(b)(4)(A), P.L. 108-446 §614 (b)(4)(A).
[29] 20 U.S.C §1414(b)(4)(B), P.L. 108-446 §614 (b)(4)(B).
[30] 20 U.S.C. §1414(b)(5), P.L. 108-446 §614 (b)(5).
[31] 20 U.S.C. §1414(a)(2), P.L. 108-446 §614 (a)(2).
[32] 34 C.F.R. §300.300(c) (2010).
[33] 20 U.S.C. §1414(c)(5), P.L. 108-446 §614 (c)(5).

is therefore worth noting the procedures required for identifying a child with an SLD. In addition to the procedures addressed above for identifying a child with a disability, the statute and regulations allow additional procedures.[34] In general, a state must adopt criteria for determining whether a child has an SLD, and an LEA must use the state criteria.[35] The state criteria cannot require the use of a severe discrepancy between intellectual ability and achievement for determining whether a child has a specific learning disability;[36] must permit the use of a process based on the child's response to scientific, research-based intervention;[37] and may permit the use of other alternative research-based procedures for determining whether a child has an SLD.[38]

In general, the group members who determine whether a child has an SLD must include the child's parents, the child's regular education teacher, and at least one person qualified to conduct individual diagnostic examinations of children (e.g., a school psychologist, speech-language pathologist, or remedial reading teacher).[39] The group may determine that a child has an SLD if three criteria are met:[40]

---

[34] 20 U.S.C. §1414(b)(6), P.L. 108-446 §614 (b)(6), and 34 C.F.R. §300.307 through §300.311 (2010).

[35] 34 C.F.R. §300.307 (2010).

[36] 20 U.S.C. §1414(b)(6)(A), P.L. 108-446 §614 (b)(6)(A), and 34 C.F.R. §300.307(a)(1) (2010). The Senate report in considering the 2004 amendments to IDEA explains the rationale for this provision:

The committee believes that the IQ-achievement discrepancy formula, which considers whether a child has a severe discrepancy between achievement and intellectual ability, should not be a requirement for determining eligibility under the IDEA. There is no evidence that the IQ-achievement discrepancy formula can be applied in a consistent and educationally meaningful (i.e., reliable and valid) manner. In addition, this approach has been found to be particularly problematic for students living in poverty or culturally and linguistically different backgrounds, who may be erroneously viewed as having intrinsic intellectual limitations when their difficulties on such tests really reflect lack of experience or educational opportunity. S.Rept. 108-185, 108th Cong., 2d Sess. 26 (2003).

[37] 20 U.S.C. §1414(b)(6)(B), P.L. 108-446 §614 (b)(6)(B).

[38] 34 C.F.R. §300.307(a)(3)(2010). In ED's analysis of comments and changes to the final regulations at 71 Fed. Reg. 46648 (August 14, 2006), ED elaborates on this criterion by stating: "For example, a state could choose to identify children based on absolute low achievement and consideration of exclusionary factors as one criterion for eligibility. Other alternatives might combine features of different models for identification."

[39] 34 C.F.R. §300.308 (2010).

[40] 34 C.F.R. §300.309(a) (2010).

- The child does not achieve adequately for the child's age or meet state-approved grade-level standards in one or more of eight areas[41] when provided with learning experiences and instruction appropriate for the child's age or state-approved grade-level standards.
- The child either does not make sufficient progress to meet age or state-approved grade-level standards in one or more of the eight areas when using a process based on the child's response to scientific, research-based intervention; or the child exhibits a pattern of strengths and weaknesses in performance, achievement, or both, relative to age, state-approved grade-level standards, or intellectual development that is determined by the group to be relevant to the identification of an SLD.
- If the child is found to have an SLD, it is not primarily the result of a visual, hearing, or motor disability; intellectual disability; emotional disturbance; cultural factors; environmental or economic disadvantage; or limited English proficiency.

To ensure that underachievement in a child suspected of having an SLD is not due to lack of appropriate instruction in reading or math, the group must consider, as part of the evaluation, (1) data that demonstrate that prior to, or as a part of, the referral process, the child was provided appropriate instruction in regular education settings, delivered by qualified personnel; and (2) data-based documentation of repeated assessments of achievement at reasonable intervals, reflecting formal assessment of student progress during instruction, which was provided to the child's parents.[42]

If prior to a referral for an evaluation, a child has not made adequate progress after an appropriate period of time when provided instruction, an LEA must promptly request parental consent to evaluate the child.[43] The

---

[41] These eight areas are oral expression, listening comprehension, written expression, basic reading skill, reading fluency skills, reading comprehension, mathematics calculation, and mathematics problem solving.

[42] 34 C.F.R. §300.309(b) (2010).

[43] 34 C.F.R. §300.309 (c). In ED's analysis of comments and changes to the final regulations at 71 Fed. Reg. 46658 (August 14, 2006), ED addresses the issue of "an appropriate period of time"

regulations also specify that the child must be observed in the child's learning environment to document the child's academic performance and behavior in the areas of difficulty.[44]

Finally, the regulations detail the specific documentation for determining eligibility for a child suspected of having an SLD.[45]

The Individualized Education Program (IEP)

FAPE is implemented through the IEP, which is the program plan that lays out how the LEA will provide special education and related services to each child with a disability. The IEP is developed by an IEP team composed of school personnel and parents. In general, the IEP team must consider the strengths of the child; the concerns of the parents; the results of the initial evaluation (or most recent evaluation); and the academic, developmental, and functional needs of the child.[46] The IEP team meets at least once a year to review the IEP to determine if goals are being met and to make necessary changes.[47] The team must meet to develop the initial IEP for a child within 30 days of determining that the child needs special education and related services. In addition, as soon as possible following the development of the IEP, special education and related services must be made available to the child in accordance with the IEP.[48]

Content of IEP[49]

Specifically, IDEA requires that the IEP include the following:

---

by stating "Instructional models vary in terms of the length of time required for the intervention to have the intended effect on a child's progress. It would not be appropriate for the Department to establish timelines ... because doing so would make it difficult for LEAs to implement models specific to their local school districts. These decisions are best left to state and local professionals who have knowledge of the instructional methods used in their school."

[44] 34 C.F.R. §300.310 (2010).

[45] 34 C.F.R. §300.311 (2010).

[46] 20 U.S.C §1414(d)(3)(A), P.L. 108-446 §614 (d)(3)(A).

[47] 20 U.S.C. §1414(d)(4), P.L. 108-446 §614 (d)(4).

[48] 34 C.F.R. §300.323(c) (2010).

[49] 20 U.S.C. §1414(d)(1)(A), P.L. 108-446 §614 (d)(1)(A).

- the child's present levels of academic achievement and functional performance;
- measurable annual goals, including academic and functional goals, designed to
    - meet the child's needs that result from the child's disability to enable the child to be involved in and make progress in the general education curriculum; and
    - meet each of the child's other educational needs that result from the child's disability;
- how the child's progress toward meeting the above annual goals will be measured and when periodic reports on the progress the child is making toward meeting the annual goals will be provided;
- the special education and related services and supplementary aids and services, based on peer-reviewed research to the extent practicable, to be provided to the child, or on behalf of the child, and the program modifications or supports for school personnel that will be provided for the child to
    - advance appropriately toward attaining the annual goals;
    - be involved in and make progress in the general education curriculum and participate in extracurricular and other nonacademic activities; and
    - be educated and participate with other children with disabilities and nondisabled children;
- the extent, if any, to which the child will not participate with nondisabled children in the regular class;
- any individual appropriate accommodations[50] that are necessary to measure the academic achievement and functional performance of the child on state and district-wide assessments; if the IEP team determines that the child will take an alternate assessment on a particular state or district-wide assessment of student achievement, the IEP should detail why the child cannot participate in the regular

[50] An accommodation is a change in instructional material or assessment practices that enable students with disabilities to reduce baiiers to learning.

assessment and why the particular alternate assessment selected is appropriate for the child;[51]

- the projected date for the beginning of the assessments and their frequency, location, and duration.

In addition, beginning not later than when the first IEP is in effect when the child is 16, and updated annually thereafter, the IEP must include appropriate measurable postsecondary goals related to training, education, employment, and, where appropriate, independent living skills and the transition services[52] needed to assist the child in reaching those goals.

The IEP Team[53]

Each child identified as a child with a disability must have an IEP developed by an IEP team. In general, the composition of the team includes

- the parents of a child with a disability;
- one or more regular education teachers, if the child is or may be participating in the regular education environment;
- one or more special education teachers;
- a representative of the LEA who is qualified to provide or supervise the provision of special education; is knowledgeable about the

---

[51] Although many students with disabilities are able to participate in the general state assessment, other students may need an alternate assessment that is tailored to their needs and allows them to more accurately demonstrate what they know and can do. For information on alternate assessments for students with disabilities, see CRS Report R40701, *Alternate Assessments for Students with Disabilities*, by Kyrie E. Dragoo.

[52] As defined at 20 U.S.C. §1401(34), P.L. 108-446 §602(34), transition services mean
a coordinated set of activities for a child with a disability that(A) is designed to be within a results-oriented process, that is focused on improving the academic and functional achievement of the child with a disability to facilitate the child's movement from school to post-school activities, including post-secondary education, vocational education, integrated employment (including supported employment), continuing and adult education, adult services, independent living, or community participation; (B) is based on the individual child's needs, taking into account the child's strengths, preferences, and interests; and (C) includes instruction, related services, community experiences, the development of employment and other post-school adult living objectives, and, when appropriate, acquisition of daily living skills and functional vocational evaluation.

[53] 20 U.S.C. §1414(d)(1)(B), P.L. 108-446 §614 (d)(1)(B).

general education curriculum; and is knowledgeable about the availability of resources of the LEA;

- an individual who can interpret the instructional implications of evaluation results;
- at the discretion of the parent or the agency, other individuals who have knowledge or special expertise regarding the child, including related services personnel, as appropriate; and
- whenever appropriate, the child with a disability.[54]

Special Education and Related Services

The provision of special education and related services is a key component of FAPE. Special education means "specially designed instruction, at no cost to parents, to meet the unique needs of a child with a disability, including (A) instruction conducted in the classroom, in the home, in hospitals and institutions, and in other settings; and (B) instruction in physical education."[55] Specially designed instruction, which is delineated in the IEP, means that the content, methodology, or delivery of instruction is adapted to address the unique needs of the child that result from the child's disability. The instruction must ensure the child's access to the general curriculum, so that the child can meet the educational standards that apply to all children. While specially designed instruction is provided at no cost to parents, parents can be required to pay any incidental fees that are normally charged to nondisabled students or their parents as a part of the regular education program.[56]

In general, related services are transportation and those developmental, corrective, and other supportive services required to help a child with a disability to benefit from special education. Both the statute and federal

[54] If the purpose of an IEP meeting is to consider the postsecondary goals for the child and transition services, the LEA must invite the child to attend the meeting; 34 C.F.R. §300.321(b)(1) (2010).
[55] 20 U.S.C. §1401(29), P.L. 108-446 §602(29), and 34 C.F.R. §300.39 (2010).
[56] 34 C.F.R. §300.39(b)(1) (2010).

regulations define related services and provide a list of related services.[57] The regulations also further define the services that may be provided to a child with a disability. The list is not exhaustive; other related services could be provided to a child with a disability. Related services include the following:

- speech-language pathology and audiology services;
- interpreting services for children who are deaf, hard of hearing, or deaf-blind;
- psychological services;
- physical therapy and occupational therapy;
- recreation, including therapeutic recreation;
- social work services in schools;
- school health services and school nurse services;
- counseling services, including rehabilitation counseling;
- orientation and mobility services provided to blind or visually impaired children;
- parent counseling and training;
- medical services for diagnostic and evaluation purposes only;[58] and
- early identification and assessment of disabilities through the implementation of a formal plan for identifying a disability.

Coordinated Early Intervening Services (CEIS)

With some restrictions, LEAs may use up to 15% of their allocations[59] "to develop and implement coordinated, early intervening services, which may include interagency financing structures, for students in kindergarten

---

[57] 20 U.S.C. §1401(26), P.L. 108-446 §602(26), and 34 C.F.R. §300.34 (2010).

[58] For a discussion of the legal issues regarding medical services as a related service, see CRS Report R40690, *The Individuals with Disabilities Education Act (IDEA): Statutory Provisions and Recent Legal Issues*, coordinated by Cynthia Brown.

[59] An LEA cannot use the full 15% for CEIS when they are also reducing funds under IDEA maintenance of effort (MOE) provisions. See the discussion in this chapter on "Maintenance of Effort (MOE)" for further explanation.

through grade 12 (with a particular emphasis on students in kindergarten through grade 3) who have not been identified as needing special education or related services but who need additional academic and behavioral support to succeed in a general education environment."[60] CEIS may not, however, delay an appropriate evaluation of a child suspected of having a disability.[61]

In its analysis of comments and changes to the final regulations, ED discusses the potential benefits of CEIS as follows:

> The authority to use some Part B funds for early intervening services has the potential to benefit special education, as well as the education of other children, by reducing academic and behavioral problems in the regular educational environment and reducing the number of referrals to special education that could have been avoided by relatively simple regular education interventions.[62]

LEAs may use CEIS funds for both professional development for teachers and other school staff and for educational and behavioral evaluations, services, and supports to students.[63] Funds may also be used to carry out CEIS that are aligned with activities funded by, and carried out under, the Elementary and Secondary Education Act of 1965 (ESEA) if the funds supplement, and do not supplant, ESEA funds.[64]

A state must require an LEA to use up to 15% of its funds for CEIS if the state has determined through statutorily required data collection that

---

[60] 20 U.S.C. §1413(f), P.L. 107-110 §613(f). Coordinated Early Intervening Services (CEIS), also referred to in statute as Early Intervening Serving (EIS), should not be confused with Early *Intervention* Services (EIS) authorized under Part C of IDEA. Part C, EIS, defined in Section 632(4), is for infants and toddlers with disabilities, while Part B CEIS is for students who are not currently identified as having disabilities but need additional support to succeed in a general education environment. (A student could receive CEIS if he or she had previously received special education, but is not currently identified as needing it. 71 Fed. Reg. 46626 (August 14, 2006) and 34 C.F.R. §300.226 (2010)).

[61] 34 C.F.R. §300.226 (c) (2010).

[62] 71 Fed. Reg. 46626-46627 (August 14, 2006).

[63] For more information on CEIS, see U.S. Department of Education, "Memorandum: Coordinated Early Intervening Services (CEIS) Under Part B of the Individuals with Disabilities Education Act (IDEA)," July 28, 2008, http://www2.ed.gov/policy/speced/guid/idea/ceis-guidance.pdf.

[64] 20 U.S.C §1413(f)(5), P.L. 107-110 §613(f)(5).

"significant disproportionality"[65] based on race and ethnicity is occurring with respect to the identification of children with disabilities; their placement in particular education settings; and the incidence, duration, and type of disciplinary actions, including suspensions and expulsions.[66] The funds are to be used to provide CEIS "to serve children in the LEA, particularly, but not exclusively, children in those groups that were significantly overidentified."[67]

Response to Intervention (RTI)

One way that coordinated early intervening services are provided is through an approach called Response to Intervention (RTI). RTI "is a multi-level framework to maximize student achievement by providing support to students at risk for poor learning outcomes."[68] While there are many models of RTI, ED notes that

> the core characteristics that underpin all RTI models are: (1) students receive high quality research-based instruction in their general education setting; (2) continuous monitoring of student performance; (3) all students are screened for academic and behavioral problems; and (4) multiple levels (tiers) of instruction that are progressively more intense, based on the student's response to instruction.
>
> For example, an RTI model with a three-tier continuum of school-wide support might include the following tiers and levels of support: (1) Tier one (Primary Intervention), for all students using high quality scientific research-based instruction in their general education setting. It would not be appropriate to use EIS funds for these activities since these students do not need additional academic and behavioral support to succeed in a general education

[65] The term "significant disproportionality" is defined by each state; 71.Fed. Reg. 46738 (August 14, 2006).

[66] 20 U.S.C. §1418(d), P.L. 108-446 §618(d).

[67] 34 C.F.R. §300.646 (b)(2) (2010).

[68] U.S. Department of Education, *Implementing RTI Using Title I, Title III, and CEIS Funds, Key Issues for Decision-maker*, p. 11, http://www2.ed.gov/programs/titleiparta/rtifiles/rti.pdf.

environment. (2) Tier two (Secondary Intervention), for specialized small group instruction of students determined to be at risk for academic and behavioral problems. It would be appropriate to use EIS funds to support these activities. (3) Tier three (Tertiary Intervention) for specialized individualized instructional/behavioral support for students with intensive needs. EIS funds could not be used if these students were currently receiving special education or related services.[69]

Highly Qualified Teachers

Each SEA must ensure that each special education teacher who teaches elementary or secondary school is "highly qualified."[70] The term "highly qualified" as defined in IDEA is linked to the definition in ESEA. In brief, ESEA requires that public school teachers of "core academic subjects"[71] obtain full state teaching certification or pass the state teacher licensing examination, or fulfill requirements in a state's charter school law for teachers in charter schools; have not had any certification requirements waived on an emergency, temporary, or provisional basis; and have a bachelor's degree.[72] IDEA modifies the ESEA definition as it applies to special education teachers.[73] IDEA requires that *all special education teachers*, whether they teach core academic subjects or not, obtain full state

---

[69] U.S. Department of Education, *Questions and Answers on Response to Intervention (RTI) and Early Intervening Services (EIS)*, January 2007, Question F-5. RTI is one type of scientific, research-based intervention used to identify students with SLD. See "Identifying and Evaluating a Child with a Specific Learning Disability (SLD)."

[70] 20 U.S.C. §1412(a)(14)(C), P.L. 108-446 §612(a)(14)(C).

[71] The term "core academic subjects" as defined in ESEA at 20 U.S.C. §7801(11), P.L. 107-110 §9101(11) means "English, reading or language arts, mathematics, science, foreign languages, civics and government, economics, arts, history, and geography." The IDEA definition of core academic subjects defined at 20 U.S.C. §1401(4), P.L. 108-446 §602(4) has the same meaning as the ESEA definition.

[72] 20 U.S.C. §7801(23), P.L. 107-110 §9101(23). For more information on ESEA requirements, see CRS Report R42127, *Teacher Quality Issues in the Elementary and Secondary Education Act*, by Jeffrey J. Kuenzi (available upon request to CRS).

[73] For more information on highly qualified teachers under IDEA, see CRS Report RL33649, *The Individuals with Disabilities Education Act (IDEA): Final Regulations for P.L. 108-446*, by Nancy Lee Jones and Ann Lordeman.

special education teaching certification or pass the state teacher licensing examination, or fulfill requirements in a state's charter school law for teachers in charter schools; have not had any certification requirements waived on an emergency, temporary, or provisional basis; and have a bachelor's degree. In addition, IDEA has specific provisions related to teachers who teach only the most severely disabled children and those who teach more than one core subject.[74]

The Educational Environment

IDEA requires that children with disabilities be educated in the least restrictive environment possible.[75] In other words, to the maximum extent that is appropriate they are to be educated with children who are not disabled. Further, special classes, separate schooling, or other removal of children with disabilities from the regular educational environment can occur only when the nature or severity of the disability of a child is such that education in regular classes with the use of supplementary aids and services[76] cannot be achieved satisfactorily. Supplementary aids and services could include such things as additional time to take tests or complete assignments, slower-paced instruction, personal aides, peer tutors, and use of a computer.

The LEA must also ensure that there is a continuum of alternate placements that includes instruction in regular classes, special classes, special schools, home instruction, and instruction in hospitals and institutions. This continuum must also make provision for supplementary services to be provided in conjunction with regular class placement.[77]

---

[74] 20 U.S.C. §1401(10), P.L. 108-446 §602(10), and 34 C.F.R. §300.18.

[75] 20 U.S.C. §1412(a)(5), P.L. 108-446 §612(a)(5). For legal issues pertaining to least restrictive environment, see CRS Report R40690, *The Individuals with Disabilities Education Act (IDEA): Statutory Provisions and Recent Legal Issues*, coordinated by Cynthia Brown.

[76] 20 U.S.C. §1401(33), P.L. 108-446 §602(33). Supplementary aids and services are defined as "aids, services, and other supports that are provided in regular education classes or other education-related settings to enable children with disabilities to be educated with nondisabled children to the maximum extent appropriate in accordance with section 612(a)(5) [Least Restrictive Environment]."

[77] 34 C.F.R. §300.115.

The specific placement decision for each child with a disability must be made by a group of persons, including the parents, and other persons knowledgeable about the child, the meaning of the evaluation data, and placement options. The child's placement must be (1) determined at least annually, (2) based on the IEP, and (3) as close to home as possible.[78]

Table 2. Percentage of Time Students Ages 6 through 21 Spend in a Regular Classroom and in Other Environments, under IDEA Part B: Fall 2015

Disability	Percentage Who Spend 80% or More of Time in a Regular Classroom	Percentage Who Spend 40%-79% of Time in a Regular Classroom	Percentage Who Spend Less than 40% of Time in a Regular Classroom	Percentage Who are Educated in Other Environments
Speech or language impairments	87%	5%	4%	4%
Specific learning disability	70%	23%	5%	2%
Other health impairments	66%	21%	9%	4%
Intellectual disabilities	17%	26%	50%	7%
Emotional disturbance	47%	17%	18%	17%
Autism	40%	18%	33%	9%
All disabilities	63%	19%	13%	5%

Source: U.S. Department of Education, EDFacts Data Warehouse (EDW): "IDEA Part B Child Count and Educational Environments Collection," 2015-2016, http://www2.ed.gov/programs/osepidea/618-data/index.html.

Notes: Percentages by disability may not add to 100% because of rounding. Total number of students is 6.05 million.

[78] 34 C.F.R. §300.116.

As with identification and evaluation, the child's parents must be notified in writing within a reasonable time before the placement.[79] If the parents disagree with the placement decision, they may use the procedural safeguards, such as the mediation and due process complaints discussed in the "Procedural Safeguards" section of this chapter.

As shown in Table 2, which contains the most recent data available, 63% of children with disabilities ages 6 through 21 spend 80% or more of their time in the regular classroom; 19% spend between 40% and 79%; 13% spend less than 40%; and 5% are educated in other environments. Other environments are a separate school, a residential facility, a private school placement by the parent, a correctional facility, and a home or hospital. Of all children with disabilities ages 6 through 21, 3% receive their education in a separate school and an additional 1.5% are parentally placed in a private school. As also shown in Table 2, 70% of children with SLDs and 87% with speech and language impairments spend 80% or more of their classroom time in the regular classroom, while 17% of children with intellectual disabilities spend 80% or more of their time in the regular classroom.

Children with Disabilities in Private Schools[80]

A child with a disability may be placed in a private elementary or secondary school by an LEA as part of an IEP if the IEP team determines that a private school placement is needed to fulfill the FAPE requirements for the child. In this situation, the private school placement is made at no cost to the parents, and the child has all of the rights of a child with a disability who is served in a public school.[81]

A child with a disability may also be unilaterally placed in a private elementary or secondary school by his or her parents.[82] In this situation, the "parentally placed" child is not entitled to FAPE, and the cost of the private

[79] 34 C.F.R. §300.503.

[80] For more information on this topic, including legal issues, see CRS Report R41678, *The Individuals with Disabilities Education Act (IDEA): Private Schools.*

[81] 20 U.S.C. §1412(a)(10)(B), P.L. 108-446 §612(a)(10)(B).

[82] 20 U.S.C. §1412(a)(10)(B), P.L. 108-446 §612(a)(10)(B).

school placement is not paid by the LEA unless a court or hearing officer makes certain findings.[83] The LEA must, however, spend a share of its IDEA funds to provide services to children enrolled with disabilities by their parents in private schools located in the LEA based on the proportion of parentally placed children to the total number of children with disabilities in the LEA.[84]

Except where there is a court order, the LEA makes the final decision about the services to be provided to parentally placed private school children.[85] In making this decision, the LEA must engage in a consultation process with the private school officials and representatives of parents.[86] The LEA is also responsible for devising a service plan for every parentally placed child with a disability receiving special education or related services from the LEA.[87]

PROCEDURAL SAFEGUARDS

Procedural safeguards[88] are provisions protecting the rights of parents and children with disabilities regarding FAPE. The various types of procedures include parental rights to

---

[83] 20 U.S.C. §1412(a)(10)(C), P.L. 108-446 §612(a)(10)(C). Specifically, an LEA could be required by a court or a hearing officer to reimburse the parents of a child with a disability who (1) previously received special education and related services from an LEA, and (2) enrolled the child in a private elementary school or secondary school without the consent of or referral by the LEA for the cost of the private school enrollment if the court or hearing officer found that the LEA had not made FAPE available to the child in a timely manner prior to the private school enrollment.

[84] 20 U.S.C. §1412(a)(10)(iii)(I), P.L. 108-446 §612(a)(10)(iii)(I). For example, if an LEA has 250 children with disabilities, 15 of whom were parentally placed in a private school, 6% of federal IDEA Part B funds (i.e., 15/250 * 100) would be spent on the group of children with disabilities in private schools in the LEA. For a more comprehensive hypothetical example, see Appendix B to 34 C.F.R. Part 300. It should be emphasized that no individual parentally placed private school child with a disability is entitled to services.

[85] 20 U.S.C. §1412(a)(10)(A)(iii), P.L. 108-446 §612(a)(10)(A)(iii).

[86] 34 C.F.R. §300.137(b) (2010).

[87] 34 C.F.R. §300.138)(b) (2010).

[88] For information on the legal issues pertaining to procedural safeguards, including burden of proof, parental rights, attorneys' and expert witness fees, see CRS Report R40690, *The Individuals with Disabilities Education Act (IDEA): Statutory Provisions and Recent Legal Issues*, coordinated by Cynthia Brown.

- inspect and review educational records;[89]
- participate in meetings related to the identification, evaluation, and educational placement of their child;[90]
- obtain an independent educational evaluation at public expense if the parent disagrees with an evaluation obtained by the LEA;[91]
- receive prior written notice in the native language of the parents when an LEA proposes to initiate or change, or refuses to initiate or change, the identification, evaluation, or educational placement of the child or the provision of FAPE to the child;[92]
- receive a procedural safeguards notice, which is a comprehensive written explanation of IDEA's legal rights and protections for children with disabilities and their parents;[93]
- resolve disputes through a mediation process;[94]
- present and resolve complaints through the due process complaint procedures, which include a right to file suit in federal district court;[95] and
- present and resolve complaints through state complaint procedures.[96]

Three of the procedural safeguards listed above pertain to dispute resolution between parents and the LEA. These are mediation, due process complaint procedures, and state complaint procedures, which are discussed below. IDEA's disciplinary provisions, discussed in this section as well, also

---

[89] 20 U.S.C. §1415(b)(1), P.L. 108-446 §615(b)(1), and 34 C.F.R. §300.501(a) (2010).

[90] 20 U.S.C. §1414(e), P.L. 108-446 §614(e), and 34 C.F.R. §300.501(b) and (c) (2010).

[91] 20 U.S.C. §1415(b)(1), P.L. 108-446 §614(b)(1), and 34 C.F.R. §300.502 (2010). If the LEA asserts that its evaluation is appropriate, it can file a due process complaint to request a hearing. If the final decision is that the agency's evaluation is appropriate, the parent still has the right to an independent education evaluation, but not at public expense.

[92] 20 U.S.C. §1415 (b)(3) and (4), P.L. 108-446 §615(b)(3) and (4), and 34 C.F.R. §300.503(a) and (c) (2010). For the statutory and regulatory provision regarding the content of the notice, see 20 U.S.C. §1415 (c)(1), P.L. 108-446 §615(c)(1), and 34 C.F.R. §300.503(b) (2010).

[93] 20 U.S.C. §1415(d), P.L. 108-446 §615(d), and 34 C.F.R. §300.504 (2010).

[94] 20 U.S.C. §1415(e), P.L. 108-446 §615(e), and 34 C.F.R. §300.506 (2010).

[95] 20 U.S.C. §1415(f) through (j), P.L. 108-446 §615(f) through (j), and 34 C.F.R. §300.507 through §300.518 (2010).

[96] 34 C.F.R. §300.151 through §300.153 (2010). State complaint procedures are not contained in the statute.

include procedural safeguards to protect the rights of children with disabilities to FAPE.

Mediation[97]

Mediation is a process of resolving disputes initiated by either the parent or LEA involving any matter under IDEA. It is a way of resolving complaints without the formal due process hearing, discussed below. Either a parent or an LEA can initiate the mediation process, which must be voluntary for each party. The mediation must be conducted by a qualified and impartial mediator who is trained in effective mediation techniques. The cost of the mediation process is borne by the state.

If the school and parent resolve a dispute through the mediation process, they must execute a legally binding agreement that is signed by the parent and a representative of the LEA. This agreement is enforceable in state or U.S. district court. Discussions that occur during the mediation process must be confidential and may not be used in any subsequent due process hearing or civil proceeding of any federal or state court.

Due Process Complaint Procedures

The due process complaint procedure begins with filing a due process complaint, which is in effect a request for a due process hearing, on matters relating to the identification, evaluation, or educational placement of a child with a disability, or the provision of FAPE to the child. Generally, unless the SEA or LEA and the parent otherwise agree, the child must remain in his or her current educational placement pending the outcome of the due process complaint procedures or of a court proceeding. This requirement is referred to as "stay put."[98]

---

[97] 20 U.S.C. §1415(e), P.L. 108-446 §615(e), and 34 C.F.R. §300.506 (2010).
[98] 20 U.S.C. §1415(j), P.L. 108-446 §615(j), and 34 C.F.R. §300.518 (2010).

Either a parent or an LEA may file a due process complaint.[99] The due process complaint must allege a violation that occurred not more than two years before the date the parent or public agency knew or should have known about the alleged action that forms the basis of the due process complaint, or, if the state has an explicit time limitation for filing a due process complaint, occurred in the time period allowed by state law.[100]

Within 15 days of receiving the due process complaint, the LEA must convene a resolution session to attempt to resolve the issues unless the parents and LEA agree to waive the session. If the issues are not resolved, the due process hearing may occur. If the complaint is not resolved through mediation, a resolution meeting, or a due process hearing, either party to the complaint can file a civil suit.[101]

The due process hearing is conducted by an impartial hearing officer.[102] The decision of the hearing officer is final, except that any party in a state where the hearing is conducted by the LEA may appeal the findings and decision to the SEA, who in turn must conduct an impartial review.

If the hearing was held in a state where the SEA conducted the hearing, then either party can file a civil lawsuit. The party filing the lawsuit has 90 days from the date of the decision of the hearing officer or, if applicable, the decision of the state review official, to file the lawsuit; or, if the state has an explicit time limitation for bringing civil action, the lawsuit must be filed in the time period allowed by state law.[103]

---

[99] 20 U.S.C. §1415(b)(7) and (8), and 20 U.S.C. §1415(c)(2), P.L. 108-446 §615(b)(7) and (8), and §615(c)(2), and 34 C.F.R. §300.507 through §300.509 (2010).

[100] There are two exceptions to this timeline. The timeline does not apply if the parent was prevented from requesting a hearing due to specific misrepresentations by the LEA that it had resolved the problem forming the basis of the due process complaint; or the LEA withheld information from the parent that was required to be provided to the parent. 20 U.S.C. §1415(b)(6), P.L. 108-446 §615(b)(6), and 34 C.F.R. §300.507(a)(2) (2010).

[101] For more detail, see the statutory and regulatory provisions at 20 U.S.C. §1415, P.L. 108-446 §615, and 34 C.F.R. Subpart E (2010).

[102] For information on conducting a due process hearing, see 20 U.S.C. §1415(f), P.L. 108-446 §615(f), and 34 C.F.R. §300.511 through §300.515 (2010). For information on the required qualifications of the hearing officer, see 20 U.S.C. §1415(f)(3), P.L. 108-446 §615(f)(3), and 34 C.F.R. §300.511(c) (2010).

[103] 20 U.S.C. §1415(g) and (i), P.L. 108-446 §615(g) and (i), and 34 C.F.R. §300.514 and §300.516 (2010).

State Complaint Procedures[104]

The IDEA regulations require each state to adopt written procedures for resolving complaints that allege LEA violations of the statute or regulations. In its analysis of comments and changes to the final regulations, ED distinguishes between the due process complaint process and the state complaint process as follows:

> The due process complaint procedures and the State complaint procedures are separate and distinct. The State complaint procedures remain a viable alternative to the due process procedures for parents to resolve disputes with public agencies in a less formal and more cost effective manner.[105]

Unlike requests for mediation or for complaints filed under due process procedures, where only a parent or an LEA can file a complaint, a state complaint can be filed by any organization or individual, including those from another state. State complaint procedures must ensure that complaints will be resolved within 60 calendar days from the date the complaint is filed unless an extension is permitted.[106]

Discipline[107]

IDEA's disciplinary provisions are intended to "balance school safety issues with the need to ensure that schools respond appropriately to a child's

---

[104] 34 C.F.R. §300.151 through §300.153 (2010).

[105] 71 Fed. Reg. 46700 (August 14, 2006).

[106] An extension of the 60-day time limit may be permitted only if exceptional circumstances exist with respect to a particular complaint or if the complainant and the LEA agree to extend the time to engage in mediation, or to engage in other alternative means of dispute resolution, if available in the state.

[107] For more information on IDEA disciplinary provisions, see CRS Report RL32753, *Individuals with Disabilities Education Act (IDEA): Discipline Provisions in P.L. 108-446*, by Nancy Lee Jones. For information on legal issues, see discussion of Honig v. Doe in CRS Report RL33444, *The Individuals with Disabilities Education Act (IDEA): Supreme Court Decisions*, by Nancy Lee Jones and Carol J. Toland.

behavior that was caused by, or directly and substantially related to, the child's disability."[108] IDEA addresses both the school's authority in disciplining students with disabilities and the rights of the students to receive FAPE. In general, a child with a disability is not immune from disciplinary procedures; however, these procedures are not identical to those for children without disabilities.[109]

If a child with a disability commits an action that would be subject to discipline, school personnel have several immediate options. These include

- removing a child from his or her current placement to another setting or suspension for up to 10 school days;[110]
- placing the child in an interim alternative education setting for up to 45 school days for situations involving weapons or drugs, or if the student has inflicted serious bodily injury on another person while at school;[111] and
- asking a hearing officer to order a child to be placed in an interim alternative educational setting for up to 45 school days if the hearing officer determines that maintaining the current placement of the child is substantially likely to result in injury to the child or others.[112]

If an LEA seeks to change the placement of a child with a disability for more than 10 days, the LEA must first determine

> (I) if the conduct in question was caused by, or had a direct and substantial relationship to, the child's disability; or (II) if the conduct in question was the direct result of the local educational agency's failure to implement the IEP.[113]

---

[108] U.S. Department of Education, *Questions and Answers on Discipline Procedures*, June 2009, https://sites.ed.gov/ idea/files/idea/policy/speced/guid/idea/discipline-q-a.pdf.

[109] 20 U.S.C. §1415(k).

[110] 20 U.S.C. §1415(k)(1)(B), P.L. 108-446 §615(k)(1)(B).

[111] 20 U.S.C. §1415(k)(1)(G), P.L. 108-446 §615(k)(1)(G).

[112] 20 U.S.C. §1415(k)(3), P.L. 108-446 §615(k)(3).

[113] To determine if the child's behavior meets either of these criteria, the LEA, the parent, and the relevant members of the IEP team must review all relevant information in the student's file, including the child's IEP, any teacher observations, and any relevant information provided by the parents; 20 U.S.C. §1415(k)(1)(E), P.L. 108-446 §615(k)(1)(E).

This determination is referred to as a "manifestation determination." The reason for the determination is IDEA's recognition "that a child with a disability may display disruptive behaviors characteristic of the child's disability and the child should not be punished for behaviors that are a result of the child's disability."[114]

If the child's behavior is not a manifestation of a disability, long-term disciplinary action such as expulsion may occur, except that educational services may not cease.[115] If the behavior is a manifestation of the disability, the IEP team must conduct a functional behavior assessment and implement a behavior intervention plan for the child, if this has not been done before.[116] If there was a behavioral intervention plan, it must be reviewed and modified as necessary to address the behavior.[117]

Except for certain circumstances involving weapons, illegal drugs, or serious bodily injury, when the conduct is a manifestation of the disability, the child must return to the placement from which he or she was removed unless the parent and the LEA agree to a change of placement as part of the modification of the behavioral intervention plan.[118] If the parent of a child with a disability disagrees with any decision regarding placement or the manifestation determination, or an LEA believes that maintaining the current placement of the child is substantially likely to result in injury to the child or others, either may request a due process hearing.[119]

Nothing in IDEA is to be construed as prohibiting an LEA from reporting a crime committed by a child with a disability to the appropriate authorities. An LEA reporting a crime committed by a child with a disability will ensure that copies of the special education and disciplinary records of the child are transmitted for consideration by the appropriate authorities to whom the agency reports the crime.[120]

---

[114] 71 Fed. Reg. 46720 (August 14, 2006).

[115] 20 U.S.C. §1415(k)(1)(C), P.L. 108-446 §615(k)(1)(C).

[116] 20 U.S.C. §1415(k)(1)(F)(i), P.L. 108-446 §615(k)(1)(F)(i). In addition, if the conduct of a child with a disability was the direct result of the LEA's failure to implement the IEP, "the LEA must take immediate steps to remedy those deficiencies"; 34 C.F.R. §300.530(e)(3) (2010).

[117] 20 U.S.C. §1415(k)(1)(F)(ii), P.L. 108-446 §615(k)(1)(F)(ii).

[118] 20 U.S.C. §1415(k)(1)(F)(iii), P.L. 108-446 §615(k)(1)(F)(iii).

[119] 20 U.S.C. §1415(k)(3)(A), P.L. 108-446 §615(k)(3)(A).

[120] 20 U.SC. §1415(k)(6), P.L. 108-446 §615(k)(6).

Funding, Expenditure Requirements, and Compliance

IDEA provides federal funding for the education of children with disabilities and imposes certain conditions for the receipt of federal funds. This section addresses state and local (1) funding allocations; (2) expenditure requirements, including maintenance of effort provisions; and (3) compliance with IDEA provisions through federal and state monitoring and enforcement requirements.

Funding

Actual and proposed grants to states are often discussed in terms of the percent of the "excess costs" of educating children with disabilities that the federal government will pay.[121] The metric for determining this excess cost is based on the national average per-pupil expenditure (APPE). In 1975, with the enactment of the Education for All Handicapped Children Act (P.L. 94-142), it was determined that the federal government would pay up to 40% of APPE to assist with this excess cost.[122] This 40% of APPE is often referred to as "full funding." In FY2017, the Part B grants to states appropriation of $12 billion provided approximately 16% of APPE.[123]

State Formula Allocations

Of the funds appropriated for IDEA, the Secretary of Education first reserves (1) not more than 1% of the appropriation for the outlying areas and

[121] The term "excess costs" is defined at 20 U.S.C. §1401 (8), P.L. 108-446 §602(8).

[122] "In 1975, when the act was originally enacted, Congress established the goal of providing up to 40% of the national average per pupil expenditure to assist states and local educational agencies with the excess costs of educating students with disabilities"; H.Rept. 108-77, p.93.

[123] CRS calculation based on unpublished data from the U.S. Department of Education.

freely associated states,[124] (2) funds for services for Indian children with disabilities,[125] and (3) not more than one-half of 1% of the appropriation up to a maximum of $25 million, adjusted for inflation, to provide technical assistance to improve the capacity of states to meet data collection requirements.[126] The remainder of the funds are allocated by a formula to the 50 states, the District of Columbia, and Puerto Rico.

If the amount available for allocations to states for a fiscal year is equal to or greater than the amount allocated to the states for the preceding fiscal year, the formula[127] first requires that each state receive a base grant, which is the amount received by the state for FY1999. The next step is to distribute 85% of the remaining funds among the states based on states' shares of total population ages 3 to 21[128] and 15% of the remaining funds based on states' shares of poor children in that age range. The third step ensures that states do not receive less than certain minimum amounts or more than certain maximum amounts.[129] If the amount available for allocation to states decreases from the prior year, any amount available for allocation to states above the 1999 level is allocated based on the relative increases in funding that the states received between 1999 and the prior year. If there is a decrease below the amount allocated for 1999, each state's allocation is ratably reduced from the 1999 level.[130]

---

[124] 20 U.S.C. §1411(b)(1), P.L. 108-446 §616(b)(1). The outlying areas are defined in §602(22) as the "United States Virgin Islands, Guam, American Samoa, and the Commonwealth of the Northern Mariana Islands." Freely associated states are defined in §611(b)(3) as "the Republic of the Marshall Islands, the Federated States of Micronesia, and the Republic of Palau."

[125] The statute at §611(b)(2) reserves 1.226% of the Part B appropriation for the Department of the Interior's Bureau of Indian Education (BIE) schools; however, this percentage has been overridden since FY2002 through the appropriations process, which has provided annual increases for BIE schools based on the rate of inflation. For example, see the language in the Special Education account in Title III of Division H of P.L. 113-76 (Consolidated Appropriations Act, 2014).

[126] 20 U.S.C. §1411(c), P.L. 108-446 §616(c).

[127] 20 U.S.C. §1411(d), P.L. 108-446 §616(d).

[128] These age ranges for this population vary from state to state depending on the age range for which each state makes FAPE available.

[129] 20 U.S.C. §1411(d)(3)(B) and 20 U.S.C. §1411(a)(2)(B), P.L. 108-446 §616(d)(3)(B) and P.L. 108-446 §616(a)(2)(B).

[130] 20 U.S.C. §1411(d)(4), P.L. 108-446 §611(d)(4).

State-Level Activities

A state may reserve funds from their grants for administration[131] and for a variety of other statewide activities. These include two mandatory activities: (1) monitoring, enforcement, and complaint investigation, and (2) establishing and maintaining a parental mediation process.[132] Other allowable state-level activities include improving the use of technology in the classroom, developing transition programs, and assisting LEAs in meeting personnel shortages.[133] In addition, for the purpose of assisting LEAs in addressing the needs of high-need children (i.e., children who require expensive services, including certain medical expenses), states may establish a risk pool or "high cost" fund. If a state chooses to establish a risk pool, it may use 10% of the funds it reserved for state-level activities.[134] States using a risk pool must develop and annually review a state plan in which the state determines which children with disabilities are high need, sets out the procedures by which LEAs participate in the risk pool, and determines how funds are distributed.[135] Funds distributed from the risk pool must only pay for "direct special education and related services" for high need children with disabilities[136] and may not be used for legal fees or related costs.[137] If some funds reserved for the risk pool are not distributed for

---

[131] 20 U.S.C. §1411(e)(1), P.L. 108-446 §611(e)(1). The amount that a state may reserve for administration is up to the greater of the maximum amount the state could reserve from FY2004 funds, or $800,000, increased by the Secretary for inflation as reflected by the Consumer Price Index for All Urban Consumers.

[132] 20 U.S.C. §1411(e)(2)(B), P.L. 108-446 §611(e)(2)(B).

[133] 20 U.S.C. §1411(e)(2)(C), P.L. 108-446 §611(e)(2)(C).

[134] 20 U.S.C. §1411(e)(3), P.L. 108-446 §611(e)(3). The percentage of a state's allocation that a state may reserve for state-level activities depends on the amount a state uses for state administration and whether or not the state uses a risk pool. A state that uses a risk pool can set aside 10.5% for state level activities if it uses $850,000 or less for state administration, or 10% if it uses $850,000 or more for state administration A state that does *not* use a risk pool can set aside 9.5% for state level activities if it uses $850,000 or less for state administration, or 9% if it uses $850,000 or more for state administration. For FY2007 and each subsequent fiscal year, each state may reserve the maximum amount the state was eligible to reserve in FY2006, cumulatively adjusted by the rate of inflation as reflected by the Consumer Price Index for All Urban Consumers. See 20 U.S.C. §1411(e)(2)(A), P.L. 108-446 §611(e)(2)(A).

[135] 20 U.S.C. §1411(e)(3)(C), P.L. 108-446 §611(e)(3)(C).

[136] 20 U.S.C. §1411(e)(3)(D)(iii), P.L. 108-446 §611(e)(3)(D)(iii).

[137] 20 U.S.C. §1411(e)(3)(E), P.L. 108-446 §611(e)(3)(E).

services for high-need children, they are to be distributed to LEAs according to the substate formula.[138]

LEA Formula Allocations

Funds remaining after funds for state-level activities are set aside are distributed to LEAs based on a formula similar to the state formula. Like the state formula, LEAs are first allocated base grants. Also similar to the state formula, 85% of the remaining funds is allocated based on LEAs' shares of public and private school enrollment and 15% of the remaining funds is allocated based on shares of children living in poverty, as determined by the SEA. There is no minimum or maximum grant.[139]

State and LEA Expenditure Requirements

IDEA state and LEA expenditure requirements are aimed at increasing overall educational spending, rather than substituting federal funds for education spending at the state and local levels. Maintenance of effort (MOE) provisions basically require that a state or an LEA not reduce its support for special education and related services below the level of support it provided the previous fiscal year. Supplement, not supplant (SNS) requirements generally prohibit a state or LEA from using IDEA grants to provide services, purchase equipment, etc., that state, local, or other federal funds currently provide or purchase or, in the absence of the IDEA funds, that those other funds would have provided or would have purchased.

Maintenance of Effort (MOE)

In general, a state may not reduce the amount of its financial support for special education and related services for children with disabilities below the amount of that support for the preceding fiscal year.[140] In any fiscal year

---

[138] 20 U.S.C. §1411(e)(3)(I), P.L. 108-446 §611(e)(3)(I).

[139] 20 U.S.C. §1411(f), P.L. 108-446 §611(f).

[140] 20 U.S.C. §1412(a)(18)(A), P.L. 108-446 §612(a)(18)(A).

in which a state does not meet this MOE requirement, the Secretary of Education is required to reduce the state's subsequent year grant by the same amount by which the state fails to meet the requirement.[141] The Secretary may grant a waiver for one fiscal year at a time in the case of "exceptional or uncontrollable circumstances" such as a natural disaster or a "precipitous and unforeseen decline in the financial resources of the state."[142] In addition, waivers can be granted if the state can provide "clear and convincing evidence" that FAPE is available for all children with disabilities.[143] If a state does not meet its MOE requirement for any year, including any year for which the state was granted a waiver, the state financial support required in future years is not reduced. That is, the state must provide the amount that would have been required in the absence of failing to meet MOE in the previous year.[144]

LEAs may use IDEA funds only for the excess costs[145] of educating children with disabilities, and may not reduce the level of expenditures for the education of children with disabilities made by the LEA from local funds below the level of those expenditures for the preceding fiscal year.[146] In general, the SEA must determine that an LEA meets this requirement (for purposes of establishing the LEA's eligibility for an award for a fiscal year). If the LEA assures the SEA that it will provide at least the same total or per capita amount from either local funds only or a combination of state and local funds for the most recent prior year for which the data are available, then the LEA would be eligible for funds.[147] IDEA specifies in statute four circumstances in which an LEA may legally reduce its local expenditures. These are in cases of

---

[141] 20 U.S.C. §1412(a)(18)(B), P.L. 108-446 §612(a)(18)(B).
[142] 20 U.S.C. §1412(a)(18)(C)(i), P.L. 108-446 §612(a)(18)(C)(i).
[143] 20 U.S.C. §1412(a)(18)(C)(ii), P.L. 108-446 §612(a)(18)(C)(ii).
[144] 20 U.S.C. §1412(a)(18)(D), P.L. 108-446 §612(a)(18)(D).
[145] For information on how an LEA calculates its excess costs, see Appendix A to Part 300, 34 C.F.R.
[146] 20 U.S.C. §1413(a)(2)(A), P.L. 108-446 §613(a)(2)(A).
[147] 34 C.F.R. §300.203(b) (2010). In practice, the MOE requirement is based on a comparison of non-federal expenditures for special education services for pupils with disabilities in the preceding fiscal year to those for the second preceding fiscal year since that would be the most recently available data.

> (1) voluntary departure, by retirement or otherwise, or departure for just cause, of special education personnel; (2) a decrease in the enrollment of children with disabilities; (3) the termination of the obligation of the agency ... to provide a program of special education to a particular child with a disability that is an exceptionally costly program ...; or (4) the termination of costly expenditures for long-term purchases, such as the acquisition of equipment or the construction of school facilities.[148]

The regulations establish a fifth circumstance under which an LEA may reduce its local expenditures. If a state establishes a risk pool (i.e., high cost fund) and the state assumes the costs associated with "high cost" children in the LEA, the LEA may reduce its expenditures.[149]

In addition, with some exceptions, an LEA may reduce its local expenditures in certain fiscal years in which its federal allocation exceeds the amount received in the previous fiscal year by not more than 50% of the excess amount.[150] These funds must be used to carry out activities authorized under ESEA.[151] Exceptions include the following: (1) the state is required to prohibit an LEA from reducing its MOE if the SEA has taken responsibility for providing FAPE in the LEA because the LEA is unable to establish and maintain programs of FAPE, or the state has taken action against the LEA under IDEA's enforcement provisions;[152] (2) if in its annual determination on the performance of LEAs, a state determines that an LEA does not meet requirements (i.e., the LEA needs assistance, intervention, or substantial intervention), the state must prohibit the LEA from reducing its MOE;[153] and (3) the amount of funds expended by an LEA for CEIS[154] must count toward the maximum amount of the reduction in expenditures the LEA may

---

[148] 20 U.S.C. §1413(a)(2)(B), P.L. 108-446 §613(a)(2)(B).

[149] 34 C.F.R. §300.204(e) (2010). See, also, the discussion in the report on "State-Level Activities."

[150] 20 U.S.C. §1413(a)(2)(C)(i), P.L. 108-446 §613(a)(2)(C)(i).

[151] 20 U.S.C. §1413(a)(2)(C)(ii), P.L. 108-446 §613(a)(2)(C)(ii).

[152] 20 U.S.C. §1413(a)(2)(C)(iii), P.L. 108-446 §613(a)(2)(C)(iii).

[153] 20 U.S.C. §1416(f), P.L. 108-446 §616(f). See the section in this chapter on "Enforcement" for more information on the federal and state performance determinations. Also, see U.S. Department of Education, *Modifications to Questions in the April 2009 Guidance on the Individuals with Disabilities Education Act, Part B, April 13, 2009*, D-7.

[154] For information on CEIS, see the section of this chapter on "Coordinated Early Intervening Services (CEIS)".

make.[155] Consequently, any LEA that is required to use 15% of its allocation on CEIS because the state has determined that "significant disproportionality"[156] based on race and ethnicity is occurring would be prohibited from reducing its MOE.[157]

Supplement, Not Supplant

Both states and LEAs must use IDEA funds to supplement state, local, and other federal funds and not to supplant them.[158] As with the state MOE requirement, the Secretary of Education has authority to grant a waiver of the state-level SNS requirement if the state provides "clear and convincing evidence" that all children with disabilities in the state have FAPE available.[159] If an LEA (or state) maintains its level of local, or state and local, expenditures for special education and related services from year to year, then the LEA has met its MOE and SNS requirements. There are no SNS or MOE waiver provisions for LEAs.[160]

Compliance

Monitoring

The Secretary monitors the implementation of IDEA through the oversight of states' required general supervision of the implementation of IDEA requirements, and through the states' required state performance plans (SPP).[161] These plans evaluate a state's efforts to implement the

---

[155] 20 U.S.C. §1413(a)(2)(C)(iv), P.L. 108-446 §613(a)(2)(C)(iv).

[156] For information on "significant disproportionality," see the section of this chapter on "Coordinated Early Intervening Services (CEIS)."

[157] U.S. Department of Education, *Modifications to Questions in the April 2009 Guidance on the Individuals with Disabilities Education Act, Part B, April 13, 1009*, D-7. The amount of funds an LEA uses for CEIS for reducing the MOE in years when there is an increase in the LEA allocation is interrelated. The decision about one use will affect the amount of funds available for the other use. For information on the interaction of CEIS and MOE, see Appendix D to Part 300, 34 C.F.R.

[158] 20 U.S.C. §1412(a)172)(C), P.L. 108-446 §613(a)(17)(C).

[159] Ibid. See 34 C.F.R. §300.164 for standards for applying for this waiver.

[160] U.S. Department of Education, *Guidance: Funds for Part B of the Individuals with Disabilities Education Act made Available Under the American Recovery and Reinvestment Act of 2009*, April 2009, C-6.

[161] 20 U.S.C. §1416(a)(1)(A), P.L. 108-446 §616(a)(1)(A).

requirements and purposes of IDEA and describe how the state will improve implementation.[162] The Secretary must enforce IDEA[163] and must also require states to monitor and enforce the implementation of IDEA by LEAs.[164] The primary focus of federal and state monitoring is on improving educational results and functional outcomes for all children with disabilities and ensuring that states meet IDEA program requirements.[165] IDEA specifies three priority areas that are to be monitored by the Secretary regarding states, and by states regarding LEAs, using quantifiable indicators to measure performance. These three monitoring priorities are:

- provision of a free appropriate public education in the least restrictive environment;
- state exercise of general supervisory authority, including child find, effective monitoring, the use of resolution sessions, mediation, voluntary binding arbitration, and a system of transition services; and
- disproportionate representation of racial and ethnic groups in special education and related services, to the extent the representation is the result of inappropriate identification.[166]

As part of an SPP,[167] each state must establish measurable and rigorous targets for the indicators established by the Secretary in the three priority areas.[168] Each state must use the targets established in its SPP and the three priority areas to analyze the performance of each LEA in the state.[169] In addition, each state must report annually to the Secretary on the state's

[162] 20 U.S.C. §1416(b)(1)(A), P.L. 108-446 §616(b)(1)(A).
[163] 20 U.S.C. §1416(a)(1)(B), P.L. 108-446 §616(a)(1)(B).
[164] 20 U.S.C. §1416(a)(1)(C), P.L. 108-446 §616(a)(1)(C).
[165] 20 U.S.C. §1416(a)(2), P.L. 108-446 §616(a)(2).
[166] 20 U.S.C. §1416(a)(3), P.L. 108-446 §616(a)(3). Each state must have in effect policies and procedures designed to prevent the inappropriate over-identification or disproportionate representation by race and ethnicity of children as children with disabilities (20 U.S.C. §1412(a)(24), P.L. 108-446 §612(a)(24)).
[167] Each state must review its SPP at least once every six years and amendments must be submitted to the Secretary; 20 U.S.C. §1416(b(1)(C), P.L. 108-446 §616(b)(1)(C).
[168] 34 C.F.R. §300.601(a)(3) (2010).
[169] 20 U.S.C. §1416(b)(2)(C)(i), P.L. 108-446 §616(b)(2)(C)(i).

performance under the SPP.[170] Annual state reporting of performance on the SPP indicators is done through the Annual Performance Report (APR).[171] The state must report annually to the public on the performance of each LEA.[172] This annual report must be made as soon as practicable, but no later than 120 days following the state's submission of its APR to the Secretary.[173] The state must also make available through public means the state's SPP, APR, and the state's annual report on the performance of each LEA in the state. At a minimum, the state must post these items on the SEA's website and distribute them to the media and through public agencies.[174]

Enforcement

Based on the information provided by the state in the SPP, information from monitoring visits, and any other public information made available, the Secretary shall determine annually if the state

- meets the requirements and purposes of IDEA Part B,
- needs assistance in implementing the requirements of IDEA Part B,
- needs intervention in implementing the requirements of IDEA Part B, or
- needs substantial intervention in implementing the requirements of IDEA Part B.

If the Secretary makes a determination that a state needs intervention or substantial intervention, the Secretary must provide notice and an opportunity for a hearing.[175]

If the Secretary determines that a state does not meet requirements, IDEA specifies a number of enforcement actions depending on the Secretary's specific determination. These actions range from advising the state of available sources of technical assistance, to requiring the state to

---

[170] 20 U.S.C. §1416(b)(2)(C)(ii)(II), P.L. 108-446 §616(b)(2)(C)(ii)(II).
[171] 20 U.S.C. §1453(d), P.L. 108-446 §653(d).
[172] 20 U.S.C. §1416(b)(2)(C)(ii)(I), P.L. 108-446 §616(b)(2)(C)(ii)(I).
[173] 34 C.F.R. §300.602(b)(i)(A) (2010).
[174] 34 C.F.R. §300.602(b)(i)(B) (2010).
[175] 20 U.S.C. §1416(d), P.L. 108-446 §616(d).

prepare a corrective action plan, to withholding, in whole or in part, further IDEA funds to the state. Prior to withholding any funds, the Secretary must provide notice and an opportunity for a hearing.[176] Whenever a state receives notice that the Secretary is proposing to take an enforcement action, the state must, at a minimum, post a notice of the pendency of an action on the SEA's website and distribute the notice to the media and through public agencies.[177]

In its analysis of comments and changes in the regulations, ED notes that

> Neither the Act nor these regulations require SEAs to publicly report on enforcement actions taken against LEAs in the State. The decision to report to the public on enforcement actions imposed on an LEA is best left to each State to decide because individual LEA circumstances vary across each State and no one set of requirements is appropriate in every situation ... However, in the interest of transparency and public accountability, the Department encourages States, where appropriate, to report to the public on any enforcement actions taken against LEAs.[178]

The state must make the same four determinations about LEAs that the Secretary makes about the states.[179] In its analysis of comments and changes in the regulations, ED comments that "States should have some discretion in making annual determination on the performance of their LEAs and, therefore, [ED] decline[s] to establish, in regulation, a uniform process for making annual determinations." ED further notes that it has advised states that in making determinations, they must consider (1) LEA performance on SPP compliance indicators,[180] (2) whether data submitted by an LEA are

---

[176] 20 U.S.C. §1416(e), P.L. 108-446 §616(e).

[177] 34 C.F.R. §300.606 (2010). The Secretary also posts the annual determination letters typically issued in June of each year to each state, Puerto Rico, the District of Columbia, and outlying areas on its website at http://www2.ed.gov/fund/ data/report/idea/partbspap/allyears.html.

[178] 71 Fed. Reg. 73203 (August 14, 2006).

[179] 20 U.S.C. §1416(a)(1)(C), P.L. 108-446 §616(a)(1)(C)(ii), and 34 C.F.R. §300.600(a)(2) (2010).

[180] Compliance indicators include, among others, the percent of districts with disproportionate representation of racial and ethnic groups in special education and related services that is the result of inappropriate identification, the percent of children with parental consent to evaluate who were evaluated and had eligibility determined within 60 days (or a state established timeframe), and a general supervision system (including monitoring, complaints, hearings, etc.)

valid and reliable for each indicator, (3) LEA-specific audit findings, and (4) an uncorrected noncompliance from any source. In addition, ED has advised states to consider performance on results indicators, such as an LEA's graduation and dropout rates or the participation rate of students with disabilities in state assessments.[181] However, the consideration of performance indicators in LEA determinations is not required.

The regulations stipulate the specific enforcement mechanisms that a state must use if the LEA does not meet requirements.[182] These mechanisms include a range of actions and are similar to those that the Secretary must use for state enforcement.[183] The regulations also require that when a state identifies LEA noncompliance with IDEA, it must ensure that the noncompliance is corrected as soon as possible, and no later than one year after the state's identification of the noncompliance.[184]

APPENDIX A. STRUCTURE OF IDEA

Part A: General Provisions

Part A includes congressional findings pertinent to the act, the purposes of the act, and definitions. The definitions included in Part A are of critical importance in interpreting the requirements of the act. These definitions include, among others, definitions of child with a disability, specific learning disability, free appropriate public education, core academic subjects, highly qualified, individualized education program, local educational agency,

---

that identifies and corrects noncompliance as soon as possible but no later than one year from identification.

[181] 73 Fed. Reg. 73021 (August 14, 2006).

[182] 34 C.F.R. §300.600(a)(3), and 34 C.F.R. §300.800 (2010).

[183] Neither the statute nor the regulations require that states permit LEAs to appeal a state decision. According to ED's guidance *Questions and Answers on Monitoring, Technical Assistance, and Enforcement*, C-11, "Whether a State's determination about an LEA's performance may be appealed is a State decision."

[184] 34 C.F.R. §300.600(e) (2010).

related services, special education, supplementary aids and services, transition services, and excess costs. These terms have been defined throughout the body of this chapter.

Part B: Assistance for Education of All Children with Disabilities

Part B provides federal funding for the education of children with disabilities and requires, as a condition for the receipt of such funds, the provision of a free appropriate public education (FAPE) to children with disabilities between the ages of 3 and 21. School districts must identify, locate, and evaluate all children with disabilities, regardless of the severity of their disability, to determine which children are eligible for special education and related services. Each child receiving services has an Individualized Education Program (IEP), created by an IEP team, delineating the specific special education and related services to be provided to meet his or her needs. The statute also contains procedural safeguards, which are provisions to protect the rights of parents and children with disabilities to ensure the provision of FAPE.

Section 619 of IDEA Part B authorizes grants to states for preschool programs serving children with disabilities ages three to five. Since Part B grants to states are used to serve children with disabilities as young as three years of age (as well as school-age children), Section 619 is not so much a separate program as it is supplementary funding for services to this age group. In general, the provisions, requirements, and guarantees under the grants to states program that apply to school-age children with disabilities also apply to children in this age group. As a result, Section 619 is a relatively brief section of the law and deals mostly with the state and substate funding formulas for the grants and state-level activities.

Part C: Infants and Toddlers with Disabilities

The general purpose of Part C is to aid each state in creating and maintaining "a statewide, comprehensive, coordinated, multidisciplinary, interagency system that provides early intervention services for infants and toddlers with disabilities and their families."[185] Services focus on children from birth through age two who are experiencing or have a high probability of experiencing "developmental delay" (as defined by the state) with respect to physical, mental, or other capacities, and on their families.[186] Services are detailed for each child and his or her family in an Individualized Family Service Plan (IFSP). Services are to be provided, to the maximum extent feasible, in "natural environments," including the home, with other infants and toddlers who are not disabled. States are required to identify a state lead agency, which might be the state educational agency (SEA) but could be other state agencies, to coordinate the program.

Part D: National Activities to Improve Education of Children with Disabilities[187]

Part D authorizes competitive grants to improve the education of children with disabilities in three areas: (1) state personnel development (Subpart 1); (2) personnel preparation, technical assistance, model demonstration projects, and dissemination of information (Subpart 2); and (3) support to improve results for children (Subpart 3).

---

[185] 20 U.S.C. §1431(b)(1), P.L. 108-446 §631(b)(1).

[186] Under certain circumstances, children with disabilities age three and over may continue to receive Part C early intervention services until they are eligible to enter kindergarten; 20 U.S.C. §14345(c), P.L. 108-446 §635(c).

[187] In addition to the statutory provisions in Part D, see the following for more information on these activities: U.S. Department of Education, *Fiscal Year 2018, Budget Summary*, pp. 17-18; and U.S. Department of Education, *Guide to U.S. Department of Education Programs,2012*, pp. 239-247.

- Under Subpart 1, competitive grants are made to SEAs for state personnel development grants to assist SEAs "in reforming and improving their systems for personnel preparation and professional development in early intervention, educational, and transitions services ..."[188]
- Under Subpart 2, competitive grants are made to entities such as SEAs, local education agencies (LEAs),[189] institutions of higher education (IHEs), and nonprofit organizations for personnel development to help ensure that there are adequate numbers of personnel with skills and knowledge needed to help children with disabilities succeed,[190] for technical assistance and dissemination of material based on knowledge gained through research and practice,[191] and for studies and evaluations.[192]
- Under Subpart 3, competitive grants are made to nonprofit organizations for parent training and information centers, which provide parents of children with disabilities with needed training and information to work with professionals in meeting the early intervention and special education needs of their children.[193] Also, under Subpart 3, competitive grants are made to entities such as SEAs, LEAs, IHEs, and nonprofit organizations for research, development, and other activities that promote the use of technology in providing special education and early intervention services.[194]

---

[188] 20 U.S.C. §1451(a), P.L. 108-446 §651(a).

[189] The term "local educational agency" means "a public board of education or other public authority legally constituted within a State for either administrative control or direction of, or to perform a service function for, public elementary schools or secondary schools in a city, county, township, school district, or other political subdivision of a State, or for such combination of school districts or counties as are recognized in a State as an administrative agency for its public elementary schools or secondary schools." 20 U.S.C. §14011(19), P.L. 108-446 §601(19). The term "school district" is often used instead of local educational agency.

[190] 20 U.S.C. §1462, P.L. 108-446 §662.

[191] 20 U.S.C. §1463, P.L. 108-446 §663.

[192] 20 U.S.C. §1464, P.L. 108-446 §664.

[193] 20 U.S.C. §1471, §1472, and §1473, P.L. 108-446, §671, §672, and §673.

[194] 20 U.S.C. §1474, P.L. 108-446 §674.

APPENDIX B. COMMONLY USED ACRONYMS

APPE	Average Per Pupil Expenditure
APR	Annual Performance Report
CEIS	Coordinated Early Intervening Services
ED	U.S. Department of Education
ESEA	Elementary and Secondary Education Act
FAPE	Free Appropriate Public Education
IDEA	The Individuals with Disabilities Education Act
IEP	Individualized Education Program
LEA	Local Educational Agency
MOE	Maintenance of Effort
RTI	Response to Intervention
SEA	State Education Agency
SNS	Supplement, Not Supplant
SPP	State Performance Plan

ACKNOWLEDGMENTS

This chapter draws on previous reports written by Nancy Lee Jones, Legislative Attorney, and former CRS analysts Ann Lordeman and Richard N. Apling.

In: Individuals with Disabilities
Editor: Aston Delgado
ISBN: 978-1-53615-030-8

Chapter 3

The Individuals with Disabilities Education Act (IDEA), Part C: Early Intervention for Infants and Toddlers with Disabilities*

Kyrie E. Dragoo

Summary

The Individuals with Disabilities Education Act (IDEA) is a statute that authorizes grant programs that support special education services. Under the IDEA, a series of conditions are attached to the receipt of grant funds. These conditions aim to provide certain educational and procedural guarantees for students with disabilities and their families.

The grant programs authorized under the IDEA provide federal funding for special education and early intervention services for children with disabilities (birth to 21 years old) and require, as a condition for the receipt of such funds, the provision of a free appropriate public education (FAPE) (i.e., specially designed instruction provided at no cost to parents

* This is an edited, reformatted and augmented version of Congressional Research Service Publication No. R43631, dated July 30, 2018.

that meets the needs of a child with a disability) and an accessible early intervention system (a statewide system to provide and coordinate early intervention services for infants and toddlers with disabilities and their families). The IDEA also outlines and requires the use of procedural safeguards pertaining to the identification, evaluation, and placement of students in special education services that are intended to protect the rights of parents and children with disabilities. These procedures include parental rights to resolve disputes through a mediation process, and present and resolve complaints through a due process complaint procedure and through state complaint procedures.

Originally enacted in 1975, the IDEA has been the subject of numerous reauthorizations to extend services and rights to children with disabilities. The most recent reauthorization of the IDEA was P.L. 108-446, enacted in 2004. The 1986 reauthorization of the IDEA created a grants program that would provide early intervention services for infants and toddlers with disabilities and their families, what is now known as Part C, Infants and Toddlers with Disabilities.

Funding for Part B of the IDEA, Assistance for Education of all Children with Disabilities, the largest part of the act, is permanently authorized. Funding for Part C, Infants and Toddlers with Disabilities, and Part D, National Activities, was authorized through FY2011. Funding for Part C and Part D programs continues to be authorized through annual appropriations.

Part C of the IDEA authorizes a grant program to aid each state in implementing a system of early intervention services for infants and toddlers with disabilities and their families. In 2016, approximately 373,000 infants and toddlers between birth and three years old received early intervention services under Part C of the IDEA. Annual funding to each state for Part C programs is based upon the state's proportion of the number of children, birth through two years old, in the general population. In FY2018, approximately $13.4 billion was appropriated for the IDEA, $470 million of which was appropriated for Part C, representing 3.5% of total IDEA funding.

Part C requires each state to implement a public awareness program and Child Find activities to identify infants and toddlers who may be eligible for early intervention services. To be eligible for early intervention services under Part C of the IDEA, an infant or toddler must meet his or her state's definition of an infant or toddler with a disability or developmental delay. Once a child meets the IDEA's eligibility criteria, the early intervention system provides an assessment of the needs of both the child and the child's family. Early intervention coordinators then either help the family coordinate services for their child through outside service providers or directly provide early intervention services to the child and the child's family, depending on the design of the early intervention system in the state. Before a child receiving Part C services turns three years old, the child is assessed to determine whether he or she will continue receiving IDEA services, and, if so, whether the child will remain in an extended Part C service arrangement or transition into a special education preschool program funded by Section 619 of Part B of the IDEA.

INTRODUCTION

Part C (Infants and Toddlers with Disabilities) of the Individuals with Disabilities Education Act (IDEA, P.L. 108-446) authorizes a formula grant program for infants and toddlers with disabilities (ages birth through two) and their families. A general purpose of these grants is to aid states in developing and implementing "a statewide, comprehensive, coordinated, multidisciplinary, interagency system that provides early intervention services for infants and toddlers with disabilities and their families."[1] In 2016, approximately 373,000 infants and toddlers received early intervention services under Part C of the IDEA.[2]

Originally enacted in 1975 as the Education for All Handicapped Children Act, P.L. 94-142,[3] the IDEA is the main federal law that provides for the education of children and youth with disabilities from birth through age 21.[4] When first enacted, the IDEA focused on ensuring that elementary and secondary school-aged children with disabilities would be provided a free and appropriate public education (FAPE). At that time, Congress found that more than half of all children with disabilities were not receiving appropriate educational services and that 1 million children with disabilities were excluded entirely from the public school system. Further, Congress found that many public school children were prevented from having successful educational experiences because their disabilities were

---

[1] 20 U.S.C. 1431 (b)(1), P.L. 108-446.

[2] U.S. Department of Education, IDEA Section 618 Data Products: State Level Data Files, *Part C: Child Count and Settings,* 2016-17, http://www2.ed.gov/programs/osepidea/618-data/state-level-data-files/index.html#cccs.

[3] The name was changed to the Individuals with Disabilities Education Act by P.L. 101-476. The public law also substituted the phrase "children with disabilities" for the phrase "handicapped children" throughout the act.

[4] 20 U.S.C. 1400 et seq.

undiagnosed.[5] Additional factors that precipitated the enactment of P.L. 94-142 included (1) judicial decisions that found constitutional requirements existed for the education of children with disabilities, (2) the inability of states and localities to fund education for children with disabilities, and (3) the potential long-term benefits of educating children with disabilities.[6]

The IDEA is primarily thought of as the nation's special education law, and Part B, which focuses on providing special education and related services to children with disabilities between the ages of 3 and 21 years old, is the largest part of the IDEA both in terms of populations served and funding level. However, the IDEA covers more than special education. The IDEA consists of four parts. Part A contains the general provisions, including the purposes of the act and definitions. The aforementioned largest part, Part B, contains provisions relating to the education of school aged children (the grants-to-states program) and the state grants program for preschool children with disabilities (Section 619).[7] Part C, the focus of this chapter, authorizes state grants for programs serving infants and toddlers with disabilities. Finally, Part D contains the requirements for various national activities designed to improve the education of children with disabilities. *Appendix A* provides a more detailed summary of each of the four parts.

Since 1975, the IDEA has been the subject of numerous reauthorizations to extend services and rights for children with disabilities. The most recent reauthorization was P.L. 108-446 in 2004. The IDEA's 1986 reauthorization added a new part related to infants and toddlers with disabilities.[8] Known originally as Part H but later changed to Part C,[9] this addition extended IDEA programs to infants and toddlers with disabilities from birth to their third

---

[5] 20 U.S.C. §1401(b), P.L. 94-142 §601(b).

[6] For more information on each of the factors that contributed to the enactment of P.L. 94-142, congressional Members and staff may request archived CRS Report 95-669, *The Individuals with Disabilities Education Act: Congressional Intent.*

[7] For more information on funding for Part B of the IDEA, see CRS Report R41833, *The Individuals with Disabilities Education Act (IDEA), Part B: Key Statutory and Regulatory Provisions* and CRS Report R44624, *The Individuals with Disabilities Education Act (IDEA) Funding: A Primer.*

[8] 20 U.S.C. §1471, P.L. 99-457 §101, "Addition of a New Part Related to Handicapped Infants and Toddlers."

[9] The reauthorization of the IDEA in 1997 changed Part H to Part C.

birthdays, when children become eligible for services under Part B of the IDEA. In 1986, Congress recognized "an urgent and substantial need" to

- enhance the development of infants and toddlers with disabilities and to minimize their potential for developmental delay;
- reduce the educational costs to our society, including our nation's schools, by minimizing the need for special education and related services after infants and toddlers with disabilities reach school age;
- minimize the likelihood of institutionalization of individuals with disabilities and maximize the potential for their independent living in society; and
- enhance the capacity of families to meet the special needs of their infants and toddlers with disabilities.[10]

With the exception of two additions, the congressional findings are virtually unchanged in the current authorization of the IDEA. Congress now recognizes "the significant brain development that occurs during a child's first 3 years of life," as a reason Part C of the IDEA is needed, and specifies Part C's intent to "enhance the capacity of State and local agencies and service providers to identify, evaluate, and meet the needs of all children, particularly minority, low-income, inner city, and rural children, and infants and toddlers in foster care."[11]

State Requirements

All states and eligible territories are currently participating in the Part C program. In order to participate in the Part C, Grants to Infants and Families program, each state must meet the requirements contained in the current IDEA statute and regulations, which include but are not limited to

---

[10] 20 U.S.C. §1472(a), P.L. 99-457 §671(a). The findings of Congress stated in P.L. 99-457, the Education of the Handicapped Act Amendments of 1986, Part H. The reauthorization of the IDEA in 1997 changed Part H to Part C.

[11] 20 U.S.C. §1431(a)(5), P.L. 108-446 §631(a)(5).

- assuring that every eligible child and family will have early intervention available to them;
- designating a lead agency to administer and supervise the Part C program and appointing an Interagency Coordinating Council (ICC) that includes parents of infants and toddlers with disabilities, early intervention service providers, and employees of relevant state agencies to advise and assist the lead agency; and
- specifying the policies and procedures that will be implemented to ensure the required components of the comprehensive statewide early intervention system are enacted.

Lead Agency

Each state's governor is responsible for designating the agency in the state that will serve as the "lead agency" for the early intervention system. Since governors choose the agency they deem most appropriate to serve as lead agency in their states, lead agencies vary from state to state, commonly being found in Departments of Education, Health, or Human Services.[12] Other examples of agencies where a state's lead agency for the early intervention system may be located include the Department of Rehabilitation Services, Department of Public Welfare, Department of Developmental Services, and the Department of Economic Security.[13]

The lead agency is responsible both for receiving the Part C grant and for administering the Part C program. In addition, the statute requires the lead agency in each state to

[12] According to a 2016 list of 56 Part C Lead Agencies in U.S. states and territories compiled by the Early Childhood Technical Assistance Center (http://ectacenter.org/partc/ptclead.asp), 32 lead agencies are led by their state's Health Department, Department of Human Services, or Department of Health and Human Services; 13 by the Department of Education; 3 are co-led by the Departments of Health and Education; and the remaining 8 lead agencies consisted of other state agencies including Developmental Services, Economic Security, and Rehabilitation Services.

[13] Early Childhood Technical Assistance Center. (2016, October). *ECTA Center List of Part C Lead Agencies as of October 2016*. http://ectacenter.org/partc/ptclead.asp.

- identify and coordinate all available resources within the state from federal, state, local, and private sources;
- assign financial responsibility to the appropriate agencies;
- enter into formal interagency agreements that define the financial responsibility of each agency for paying for early intervention services; and
- develop procedures to ensure that both early intervention services for infants and toddlers with disabilities and dispute resolution services for families, agencies, and service providers are provided in a timely manner.

State Interagency Coordinating Council

In addition to designating the state's lead agency, the governor is responsible for appointing a state ICC to advise and assist the lead agency in various activities, including identifying and assigning financial responsibility to the appropriate agencies, promoting interagency agreements, and preparing applications and amendments for Part C. The ICC also advises and assists the state educational agency (SEA) in matters related to thc transitioning of toddlers with disabilities out of early intervention services and into preschool programs or other services, and prepares an annual report to the governor and the Secretary of Education (hereinafter referred to as the Secretary) on the status of early intervention services for infants and toddlers with disabilities and their families within the state.

In appointing members to the ICC, the Governor needs to ensure the council reasonably represents the population of the state and is comprised of members of various stakeholder groups. At least 20% of the ICC must be comprised of parents of children with disabilities, and at least one of the parent members must have a child with a disability who is younger than seven years old. Another 20% or more of the ICC must be comprised of early intervention service providers. The ICC must also contain at least one member from each of the following groups: (1) the state legislature, (2) the SEA responsible for preschool services to children with disabilities, (3) an agency involved in personnel preparation, (4) each of the state agencies involved in the provision of, or payment for, early intervention services to infants and toddlers with disabilities and their families, (5) the agency responsible for the state Medicaid program, (6) a Head Start agency or program, (7) a state agency responsible for child care, (8) the agency responsible for the state regulation of health insurance, (9) a representative designated by the Office of Coordinator for Education of Homeless Children and Youths, (10) the state child welfare agency responsible for foster care, and (11) the state agency responsible for children's mental health.[14]

SERVICES FOR INFANTS AND TODDLERS WITH DISABILITIES

Early intervention (EI) is designed to ensure that all infants and toddlers with diagnosed disabilities or developmental delays are identified and evaluated and have an individualized plan developed to meet their and their families' unique needs. This section of the report addresses (1) criteria infants and toddlers must meet to receive services under Part C of the IDEA, (2) how young children are identified and evaluated for early intervention services, and (3) the procedures for developing an individualized plan to provide services.

Infants and Toddlers with Disabilities

Part C of the IDEA defines an "infant or toddler with a disability" as a child who is experiencing a developmental delay or who because of a

[14] 20 U.S.C. §1441(b), P.L. 108-446 §641(b). The council may include other members selected by the Governor, including a representative from the Bureau of Indian Affairs (BIA), or where there is no BIA operated or BIA-funded school, from the Indian Health Service or the tribe or tribal council. Note: the BIA school system is now known as the Bureau of Indian Education (BIE). The BIE was formerly the Office of Indian Education Programs (OIEP) in the BIA. In 2006, the Secretary of the Interior moved the OIEP out of the BIA and made it an agency equivalent to the BIA, renaming it the BIE.

diagnosed condition has a high probability of experiencing a developmental delay. Thus, the key concept for receipt of early intervention services is developmental delay.[15] States are required to develop and use a "rigorous definition of the term 'developmental delay'"[16] and provide a timely and comprehensive evaluation of each child suspected of having a developmental delay, or a disability which may cause a developmental delay, in one or more of the following developmental areas:

- physical development (e.g., sitting up, rolling, crawling, or walking);
- cognitive development (e.g., processing information, learning, problem solving, thinking);
- communication development (e.g., listening, understanding, speaking);
- social or emotional development (e.g., interacting, playing, dealing with challenges);
- adaptive development (e.g., self-help, eating, dressing, adjusting to new situations).

The definition of the term "developmental delay" in Part C of the IDEA is broad, allowing each state to specify both the criteria that constitute a developmental delay in each of the aforementioned five developmental areas and the evaluation and assessment procedures to measure children's development in that area.[17] In addition to serving infants and toddlers with

---

[15] 20 U.S.C. §1432(5)(A), P.L. 108-446 §632(5)(A). In contrast, under Part B of the IDEA a child may qualify for special education under any one of 14 different disability categories: autism, deaf-blindness, deafness, developmental delay, emotional disturbance, hearing impairment, intellectual disability, multiple disabilities, orthopedic impairment, other health impairment, specific learning disability, speech or language impairment, traumatic brain injury, and visual impairment. 20 U.S.C. §1401(3)(A), P.L. 108-446 §602(3)(A).

[16] 20 U.S.C. §1435(a)(1), P.L. 108-446 §635(a)(1). Information on states' definitions of developmental delay can be found at Early Childhood Technical Assistance Center (2016). *States' Part C Rules, Regulations and Policies*, http://www.ectacenter.org/partc/statepolicies.asp.

[17] For more information on states' criteria for Part C eligibility see *Summary Table of States' and Territories' Definitions of/Criteria for IDEA Part C Eligibility*, NECTAC, the National Early Childhood Technical Assistance Center, Chapel Hill, NC, March 5, 2015, http://www.nectac.org/~pdfs/topics/earlyid/partc_elig_table.pdf.

developmental delays, states may serve infants and toddlers who are at-risk for experiencing substantial developmental delays if they do not receive early intervention services.

Accessing and Entering the Early Intervention System

In order for children to start receiving early intervention services, they must first be identified as having a disability that qualifies for services and then they must be evaluated to determine if they meet their state's criteria for services. To ensure the prompt and proper identification and evaluation of children with disabilities, each state is required to develop a public awareness program focused on early identification of infants and toddlers with disabilities. This section of the report discusses how a child enters the early intervention system, starting with the state's public awareness program and child find system, followed by the identification and evaluation process.

Pre-referral: Public Awareness Program and Child Find

The main purpose of the public awareness program is to inform parents of infants and toddlers with disabilities about the availability of early intervention services and parents of preschool-aged children about services provided under Section 619 of the IDEA.[18] Part C of the IDEA requires each state to operate a public awareness program to inform state residents about (1) early intervention services available to help eligible infants and toddlers with developmental delays or disabilities; (2) the steps to take to have an infant or toddler evaluated for early intervention eligibility; and (3) who families should contact in the early intervention system, if they have a child who may be in need of early intervention services. To this end, each state's lead agency is responsible for preparing and disseminating information on early intervention services and Section 619 to primary referral sources—those people and institutions most likely to interact with infants and toddlers

[18] 20 U.S.C. §1419, P.L. 108-446 §619. Section 619 is in Part B of the IDEA. Section 619 deals with preschool grants for children with disabilities who are three through five years old.

who may have disabilities. The Part C regulations provide a list of primary referral sources that includes

- hospitals (including prenatal and postnatal care facilities),
- physicians,
- parents of infants and toddlers (especially parents with premature infants or infants with other physical risk factors associated with learning or developmental complications),
- child care and early learning programs,
- local education agencies (LEAs),[19]
- public health facilities,
- social service agencies,
- clinics or health care providers,
- child welfare agencies, and
- homeless and domestic violence shelters.[20]

The IDEA Part C regulations require that these primary referral sources are provided with certain specific pieces of information. The state's lead agency is responsible for alerting the primary referral sources that early intervention services are available to all infants and toddlers with qualifying disabilities or developmental delays. In addition, primary referral sources must be provided with the following information:[21]

- A description of the child find system (explained in more detail in the next section of this chapter) and procedures for referring a child

---

[19] The term "local educational agency" (or LEA) means "a public board of education or other public authority legally constituted within a State for either administrative control or direction of, or to perform a service function for, public elementary schools or secondary schools in a city, county, township, school district, or other political subdivision of a State, or for such combination of school districts or counties as are recognized in a State as an administrative agency for its public elementary schools or secondary schools." 20 U.S.C. §14011(19), P.L. 108-446 §601(19). The term "school district" is often used instead of local educational agency.

[20] 34 C.F.R. §303.303.

[21] 20 C.F.R. §303.301. A list of information that primary referral sources must be provided is not contained in the statute.

under the age of three for an evaluation or early intervention services; and

- A central directory that is accessible to the general public (i.e., through the lead agency's website and other appropriate means) and includes accurate, up-to-date information about
- public and private early intervention services, resources, and experts available in the state;
- professional and other groups (including parent support, and parent training and information centers, such as those funded under the IDEA) that provide assistance to infants and toddlers with disabilities eligible under Part C of the IDEA and their families; and
- research and demonstration projects being conducted in the state related to infants and toddlers with disabilities.

In addition, the lead agency must ensure that parents of toddlers with disabilities are informed about the availability of services under Section 619 of the IDEA (i.e., services for children with disabilities who are over three years old) not fewer than 90 days prior to their child's third birthday.

Child Find

Each state must have in effect policies and procedures to ensure that all children with disabilities residing in the state who are in need of early intervention services or special education are identified, located, and evaluated. These policies and procedures are referred to in the statute as "child find."[22] The infants and toddlers covered under child find include those with disabilities who are

- homeless or wards of the state,
- Indians residing on reservations,
- suspected of having a disability, and
- highly mobile children, including migrant children.

---

[22] 20 U.S.C. §1412(a)(3), P.L. 108-446 §612(a)(3) and 20 U.S.C. §1435(a)(5), P.L. 108-446 §635(a)(5).

An infant or toddler who has been identified as having (or possibly having) a disability or a developmental delay must be evaluated before receiving early intervention services to determine whether the child is a child with a disability and to determine the developmental needs of the child.[23] Either the parent or a member of one of the primary referral sources may request an initial evaluation.[24]

Child Evaluation

When an evaluation of an infant or toddler is needed, multiple procedures must be employed, including

- administering an evaluation instrument;
- taking the child's history (including interviewing the parent);
- identifying the child's level of functioning in each
- developmental area;[25]
- gathering information from other sources such as
- family members, other care-givers, medical providers, social workers, and educators, if necessary, to understand the full scope of the child's unique strengths and needs; and
- reviewing medical, educational, or other records.

A comprehensive child find system is a key component of both Part B[26] and Part C of the IDEA. However, Part C includes several additional child find requirements specific to identifying infants and toddlers with

[23] 20 U.S.C. §1414(a), P.L. 108-446 §414(a). This subsection contains the requirements for evaluations, parental consent, and reevaluations.

[24] The LEA may refuse the parent's request for an initial evaluation if it does not suspect that the child has a disability. However, the public agency must provide written notice to the parents, consistent with 34 C.F.R. §300.503(b)(2010) and §615(c)(1) of the act, which explains, among other things, why the public agency refuses to conduct an initial evaluation and the information that was used as the basis to make that decision. The parent may challenge such a refusal by requesting a due process hearing. (71 Fed. Reg. 46636 (August 14, 2006)).

[25] The developmental areas that must be evaluated are physical development, cognitive development, communication development, social or emotional development, and adaptive development.

[26] For more information about Part B of the IDEA see CRS Report R41833, *The Individuals with Disabilities Education Act (IDEA), Part B: Key Statutory and Regulatory Provisions*.

disabilities, who due to their young age are not affiliated with the school system yet and therefore need to be identified for possible services through different mechanisms than their Part B peers. The first additional requirement of a state's Part C child find system is that it must include an efficient system for making referrals to service providers.[27] In addition, each state's child find system must provide for participation by the primary referral sources discussed in the previous section of this chapter. Finally, Part C requires the referral system to employ "rigorous standards for appropriately identifying infants and toddlers with disabilities for services ... that will reduce the need for future services."[28]

Referral Activities: Screening, Evaluations, and Assessment

Once the required components of a child find system are in place, each state has options as to how they will implement their child find system. States may choose to use screening procedures to determine which children are suspected of having disabilities, or they may choose to rely on health care workers and other primary referral sources that interact with infants and toddlers with disabilities to refer families of children with potential need of early intervention services for evaluation. In either case, the parent of a child being referred must be provided with prior written notice of their rights and provide consent before the initial screening, evaluation, or assessment of their child takes place. If the state conducts an initial screening, and that screening does not identify any potential disability or developmental delay, but the parent suspects one exists, the parent can request a full evaluation.

In conducting the evaluation, each statewide early intervention system must provide a timely, comprehensive, multidisciplinary evaluation of the functioning of each infant or toddler suspected of having a disability. In general, the lead agency must obtain informed consent from the parent before conducting an initial evaluation.[29] However, parental consent for an

---

[27] Timelines must be included in the state's system for making referrals to service providers to ensure its efficiency. 20 U.S.C. §1435, P.L. 108-446 §635 (a)(5).

[28] 20 U.S.C. §1435, P.L. 108-446 §635 (a)(5).

[29] The term "consent" is defined at 34 C.F.R. §300.9, and means, in part, that "the parent has been fully informed of all information relevant to the activity for which consent is sought, in his or

evaluation cannot be construed as consent for early intervention services or special education services.[30]

Child and Family Assessment

Assessment of the child must include:

- a review of the results of the evaluation conducted to determine the child's eligibility for EI services;
- personal observations of the child; and
- the identification of the child's needs in each of five developmental areas.[31]

Family-directed assessment must:

- be voluntary on the part of each family member participating in the assessment;
- be based on information obtained through an assessment tool and also through an interview with those family members who choose to participate in the assessment; and
- include the family's description of its resources, priorities, and concerns related to enhancing the child's development.

A child's records[32] may be used to establish eligibility (without conducting an evaluation of the child) if those records indicate that the

her native language, or other mode of communication." For more information on parental consent, see also 34 C.F.R. §300.300 (2010).

[30] In addition, at the time of the referral or parent request for evaluation, the LEA must provide the parent with the "Procedural Safeguards Notice," which is a comprehensive written explanation of IDEA's legal rights and protections for children with disabilities and their parents. See 20 U.S.C. §1415(d), P.L. 108-446 §615(d). For further information on procedural safeguards, see "Procedural Safeguards " in this chapter.

[31] The developmental areas that must be evaluated are physical development, cognitive development, communication development, social or emotional development, and adaptive development.

[32] 31 Records in this instance refers to either medical or other relevant records, 34 C.F.R. §303.321(a)(3)(i).

child's level of functioning[33] constitutes a developmental delay or that the child has a diagnosed condition that creates a high probability that the child will experience a developmental delay. For example, an infant's medical records are often used to establish eligibility for early intervention, when a baby is born prematurely or diagnosed with a disability at birth.

Once a child is determined to be a Part C eligible infant or toddler, the early intervention system must provide a multidisciplinary assessment of the unique strengths and needs of the child and identify the services appropriate to meet those needs.[34] The assessment of each infant or toddler with a disability must be conducted by qualified personnel who can identify both the child's needs and the appropriate early intervention services to meet those needs. With the parents' consent, early intervention services may start prior to the completion of the assessment.[35]

In addition to the assessment of the child, the early intervention system requires a family-directed assessment of the resources, priorities, and concerns of each child's family and identification of the supports and services necessary to enhance the family's abilities to meet the developmental needs of their infant or toddler with a disability.[36] The focus on the needs of a child's family and assessing the supports and training the family needs in order to best support their child with a disability is one of the main elements that differentiates the Part C early intervention system from the Part B special education system. Early intervention (Part C) focuses on training family members to provide the interventions and supports their child's needs in the child's natural environment (i.e., at home or in a community setting). Special education (Part B) generally provides supports and services in a school setting and rarely includes assessing the needs of or providing training for other members of the child's family.

---

[33] Levels of functioning in one or more of the developmental areas identified in the Part C definition of disability. For a discussion of the definition of disability and developmental delay in Part C of the IDEA see the earlier section of this chapter, "Infants and Toddlers with Disabilities."

[34] 20 U.S.C. §1436(a)(1), P.L. 108-446 §636(a)(1) and 34 C.F.R. §303.321(c)(1).

[35] A thorough evaluation may take several weeks, particularly if a child is being evaluated by multiple specialists (e.g., speech therapist, special education teacher, occupational therapist, physical therapist, etc.).

[36] 20 U.S.C. §1436, P.L. 108-446 §636 and 34 C.F.R. §303.321(c)(2).

The IDEA Part C family-directed assessment must be conducted by qualified personnel in order to identify the family's resources, priorities, and concerns and the supports and services necessary to enhance the family's capacity to meet the developmental needs of their infant or toddler with a disability. The family assessment and the child assessment may be conducted together or separately depending on the needs of the family. Assessments and other evaluation materials used to assess a child must be selected and administered so as not to be discriminatory on a racial or cultural basis. In addition, all assessments and evaluations of both children and their families must be provided and administered in the family's native language unless clearly not feasible to do so.[37]

INDIVIDUALIZED FAMILY SERVICES PLAN (IFSP)

Every child who is found eligible for early intervention services is required to have an individualized family services plan (IFSP) developed within a reasonable time after the assessment is completed. Like the IEP,[38] its counterpart for children with disabilities ages 3 to 21 years old, the IFSP is a plan developed by a multidisciplinary team, including the child's parents, which outlines the early intervention services the child is going to receive. However, IFSPs differ from IEPs in much the same way the early intervention assessment process differs from the special education assessment process—IFSPs focus not only on the infant or toddler's needs but also on the needs, priorities, and concerns of other family members regarding the child.

Each child's IFSP must contain the following:

---

[37] 20 U.S.C. §1414, P.L. 108-446 §614 (b)(3)(A) and §1412, P.L. 108-446 §612 (a)(6) and 34 C.F.R. §303.321(a).

[38] The Individualized Education Program (IEP) is a plan for providing an individual child with special education and related services. For more information on the IEP process and special education services for children with disabilities ages 3 to 21 years old, see CRS Report R41833, *The Individuals with Disabilities Education Act (IDEA), Part B: Key Statutory and Regulatory Provisions.*

- the infant's or toddler's present physical, cognitive, communication, social or emotional, and adaptive development levels and needs;
- the family's resources, priorities, and concerns relating to enhancing the development of the infant or toddler with a disability;
- measurable results or outcomes expected to be achieved for the infant or toddler and the family;[39]
- the specific services the infant or toddler will be receiving, including a statement of the frequency, intensity, and method of delivering services;
- a statement of the natural environments (e.g., home or community setting) in which early intervention services will be provided to the infant or toddler, or, if any services will not be delivered in a natural environment, a justification for why not;[40]
- when and where the child will receive services, and when the services are expected to begin;
- the number of days or sessions the infant or toddler will receive each service and how long each session will last;
- the name of the service coordinator overseeing the implementation of the IFSP;[41] and
- the steps to be taken to support the transition of the toddler with a disability to preschool or other appropriate services.[42]

---

[39] These include "pre-literacy and language skills, as developmentally appropriate for the child, and the criteria, procedures, and timelines used to determine the degree to which progress toward achieving the results or outcomes is being made and whether modifications or revisions of the results or outcomes or services are necessary." (20 U.S.C. §1435, P.L. 108-446 §636 (d)(3).)

[40] Natural environments are defined in the Part C regulations as "settings that are natural or typical for a same-aged infant or toddler without a disability, may include the home or community settings, and must be consistent with [other Part C provisions regarding natural environments]." (34 C.F.R. §303.26)

[41] The service coordinator must be selected "from the profession most immediately relevant to the infant's or toddler's or family's needs (or who is otherwise qualified to carry out all applicable responsibilities under this part) who will be responsible for the implementation of the plan and coordination with other agencies and persons, including transition services." (20 U.S.C. §1435, P.L. 108-446 §636 (d)(7)).

[42] 20 U.S.C. §1435, P.L. 108-446 §636 (d).

The IFSP must be fully explained to the parents, and their suggestions must be considered. In addition, a parent must give written consent for each proposed service. If a parent or guardian does not give his or her consent in writing for a particular service, the child will not receive that service.

Timeframes

The IFSP must be reviewed every six months and the child must be evaluated at least once a year to determine if the child still qualifies for Part C services and if the current IFSP is still appropriate. The IFSP can be reviewed more frequently when that is appropriate for the child or family's needs. These provisions take into account that children can learn, grow, and change quickly in a short period of time.

The timeline for all the procedures leading up to and including the writing of the IFSP is short (45 days) for the same reasons. In comparison, twice as long (90 days) can elapse from the time a parent provides permission for their child to be evaluated for Part B special education services until the time the child's initial IEP is written.[43] The Part C 45-day time clock starts running when the lead agency or early intervention services provider receives a referral about an infant or toddler with a suspected disability or developmental delay, and within that 45-day timeframe, the early intervention system must complete the steps discussed thus far to prepare the child for early intervention services

- child find,
- screening,[44]
- initial evaluation of the child,

[43] Up to 30 days is allowed for an IEP team to be convened and draft the initial IEP for a child receiving special education; and up to 60 days is allowed to evaluate a child for special education services (20 U.S.C. §1414, P.L. 108- 446 §614 (c)(i)).

[44] This step is only required in states where screening is a designated step in the early intervention process.

- initial assessments of the child and family, and
- writing the IFSP (if the child has been found eligible).[45]

There are two exceptions to the 45-day timeline: (1) if a child is referred less than 45 days prior to his or her third birthday, the lead agency is not required to evaluate the child,[46] and (2) if the parent has not provided consent to the initial screening, evaluation, or assessment of the child, despite documented, repeated attempts to obtain parental consent.

Transition/Exiting Part C

Transition services are services that help a toddler with a disability and his or her family transition from the child's early intervention program under Part C of the IDEA to the child's next program or services, or help them prepare for the end of services under the IDEA. Every toddler with a disability receiving Part C services must have a transition plan in place, at the earliest 9 months and at the latest 90 days, before their third birthday. The transition plan must outline the transition services he or she is to receive. The transition plan is part of a child's IFSP, not an additional document. The transition services outlined in the transition plan may be designed to help the toddler and his or her family (1) transition into a Part B program, (2) continue in an extended Part C program,[47] or (3) prepare for the end of services under the IDEA, if the child is no longer eligible to receive Part C or Part B services.

Each state must provide a description of the policies and procedures to be used to ensure a smooth transition for toddlers receiving early intervention services under Part C to preschool, school, other appropriate services, or out

[45] 20 U.S.C. §1436, P.L. 108-446 §636, and 34 C.F.R. §303.310.

[46] Instead, if the child may be eligible for services under Part B of the IDEA, the lead agency, with parental consent, is required to refer the child to the Part B program. 34 C.F.R. §303.209(b)(1)(iii).

[47] Part C services generally end when a child turns three, but §303.211 allows each state to develop and implement a policy in which parents can choose to continue receiving services under Part C instead of transitioning to services under Section 619 of Part B of the IDEA.

of early intervention, in the application and assurances they submit to the Secretary in order to receive Part C funds.[48] States must delineate

- procedures for the establishment of a transition plan for each child, including, when appropriate, steps to exit from the Part C program;
- descriptions of how the families of toddlers receiving early intervention services will be included in the transition plans;
- procedures that will be used to review each child's program options for the period from the child's third birthday through the remainder of the school year; and
- how the lead agency will (1) notify LEAs when each child will shortly reach the age of eligibility for preschool scrviccs under Part B; (2) convene a conference among the lead agency, the family, and the LEA, between 9 months and 90 days before the child is eligible for preschool services, to discuss any such services that the child may receive; and (3) in the case of a child who may not be eligible for preschool services, convene a conference among the lead agency, the family, and providers of appropriate services for children who are not eligible for preschool services under Part B,[49] to discuss the appropriate services that the child may receive.

Figure 1 displays the most recent state reported data on the programs or services children receiving early intervention services transition to when they turn three years old. The columns on either end of the chart (Part B eligible and Continued in Part C) represent children who were determined to continue to have disabilities or developmental delays that require IDEA intervention services. The two inner columns (Not Part B eligible and IFSP complete) represent children who no longer qualified as having a disability or developmental delay after receiving early intervention services and were transitioning out of Part C by their third birthday.

[48] 20 U.S.C. §1437, P.L. 108-446 §637 (a)(9).

[49] Examples of appropriate service providers include private speech, occupational, or physical therapists for children who continue to have some areas of weakness but who are no longer delayed enough to be eligible for IDEA mandated services.

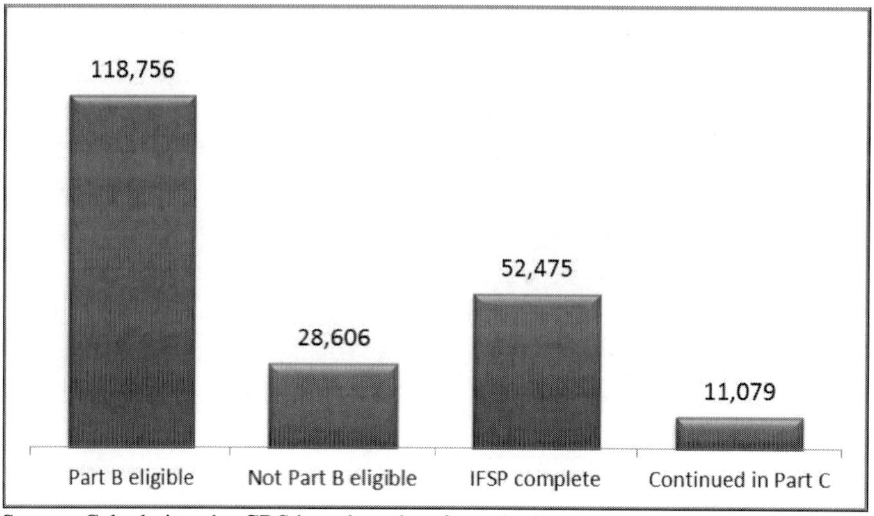

Source: Calculations by CRS based on data from the IDEA Section 618 Data Products: State Level Data Files, 2015-16 IDEA Part C Exiting, http://www2.ed.gov/programs/osepidea/618-data/state-level-data-files/index.html#ce.

Notes: Total number of children exiting Part C was approximately 326,400. This figure reflects only data on the 210,916 exiting children whose reasons for exiting included the environments they would transition to when they turned three years old. Other categories reported to the Office of Special Education Programs (OSEP) in the U.S. Department of Education but not shown here include attempts to contact unsuccessful, deceased, moved out of state, and withdrawal by parent.

"Continued in Part C" refers to children whose families requested they continue receiving Part C services when their child turned three years old, and would normally transition to Part B services. This option sometimes occurs when services are only expected to last a month or two into a child's third year, at which point they will stop receiving any IDEA (Part C or Part B) services.

Figure 1. Number of Children Who Exited Part C by Post-Exit Transition Category: 2015-2016 School Year.

Over one-third (38%) of the children represented in *Figure 1* no longer required IDEA services by the time they turned three years old. The total number of children exiting Part C in 2014-2015 was approximately 326,400. The difference between the total number and the number in *Figure 1* (approximately 115,500) was due to the exclusion of categories such as "Attempts to contact unsuccessful," "Part B eligibility not determined," and "Withdrawal by parents." If all categories were included, the percentage of students explicitly categorized as no longer requiring IDEA services by their third birthday would be 25%.

PROCEDURAL SAFEGUARDS

Procedural safeguards[50] are provisions protecting the rights of parents of infants and toddlers with disabilities and the infants and toddlers themselves regarding appropriate early intervention services. The various types of procedural safeguards include parental rights to

- inspect and review educational records;
- receive timely administrative resolution of complaints;
- maintain confidentiality of personally identifiable information;[51]
- receive prior written notice in their native language when the lead agency or an early intervention services provider proposes to initiate or change, or refuses to initiate or change, the identification, evaluation, or placement of their infant or toddler, or the provision of early intervention services to their infant or toddler;[52]
- receive a procedural safeguards notice, which is a comprehensive written explanation of the IDEA's legal rights and protections for infants and toddlers with disabilities and their parents;[53]

---

[50] 20 U.S.C. §1439, P.L. 108-446 §639, and 34 C.F.R. §303.405.

[51] This includes "the right of parents to written notice of and written consent to the exchange of such information among agencies consistent with Federal and State law," 20 U.S.C. §1439(a)(2), P.L. 108-446 §639(a)(2), and 34 C.F.R. §303.402.

[52] 20 U.S.C. §1439(a), P.L. 108-446 §639(a)(6) and (7), and 34 C.F.R. §303.421(a) and (c). For the statutory and regulatory provision regarding the content of the notice, see 20 U.S.C. §1415(c)(1), P.L. 108-446 §615(c)(1), and 34 C.F.R. §303.421(b).

[53] Part C extends procedural safeguards for children in Part B to "Procedures to protect the rights of the infant or toddler whenever the parents of the infant or toddler are not known or cannot be found or the infant or toddler is a ward of the State, including the assignment of an individual (who shall not be an employee of the State lead agency, or other State agency, and who shall not be any person, or any employee of a person, providing early intervention services to the infant or toddler or any family member of the infant or toddler) to act as a surrogate for the parents." (Part B: 20 U.S.C. §1415(d), P.L. 108-446 §615(d). Part C: 20 U.S.C. §1439(a), P.L. 108-446 §639(a)(5) and (6), and 34 C.F.R. §303.422.)

- resolve disputes through a mediation process;[54]
- determine whether they, their infant or toddler, or other family members will accept or decline any early intervention services without jeopardizing other early intervention services; and
- continue receiving[55] appropriate early intervention services for their infant or toddler, during the pendency of any proceeding or action involving a complaint filed on their family's behalf.

Prior Written Notice

The most primary of the procedural safeguards may be the right to prior written notice of any changes to a child's early intervention services. Prior written notice, delineating the list of procedural safeguards highlighted above, must be provided to parents within a "reasonable" time before the lead agency or an early intervention services provider proposes, or refuses, to initiate or change the identification, evaluation, or placement of an infant or toddler, or the provision of early intervention services to an infant or toddler with a disability.[56] If an infant or toddler is not found eligible for early intervention services, the lead agency must provide the parent with prior written notice that includes information about the parent's right to dispute the eligibility determination through dispute resolution mechanisms, such as requesting a due process hearing, mediation, or filing a state complaint.

---

[54] Part C extends "The right of parents to use mediation in accordance with section 615, except that—(A) any reference in the section to a State educational agency shall be considered to be a reference to a State's lead agency established or designated under section 635(a)(10); (B) any reference in the section to a local educational agency shall be considered to be a reference to a local service provider or the State's lead agency under this part, as the case may be; and (C) any reference in the section to the provision of a free appropriate public education to children with disabilities shall be considered to be a reference to the provision of appropriate early intervention services to infants and toddlers with disabilities." (Part B: 20 U.S.C. §1415(e), P.L. 108-446 §615(e). Part C: 20 U.S.C. §1439(a), P.L. 108-446 §639(a)(8)).

[55] "... or, if applying for initial services, shall receive the services not in dispute," §1439(b), P.L. 108-446 §639(b).

[56] 20 U.S.C. §1439, P.L. 108-446 §639 (a)(6) and 34 C.F.R. §303.421.

Mediation

Mediation[57] is a process of resolving disputes initiated by either the parent or the local service provider involving any matter under the IDEA including those under Part C. It is a way of resolving complaints without the formal due process hearing, discussed below. Either a parent or a local service provider can initiate the mediation process, which must be voluntary for each party. Mediation must be conducted by a qualified and impartial mediator who is trained in effective mediation techniques. The cost of the mediation process is borne by the state. The state cannot deny a family or service provider the opportunity for mediation. However, either party can refuse to participate in mediation, requiring the remaining party to pursue due process or state complaint procedures to resolve their dispute.

If the local service provider and parent resolve a dispute through the mediation process, they must execute a legally binding agreement that is signed by the parent and a representative of the local service provider. This agreement is enforceable in state or U.S. district court. Discussions that occur during the mediation process must be confidential and may not be used in any subsequent due process hearing or civil proceeding of any federal or state court.

Due Process Complaint Procedures

States may elect to adopt either IDEA Part B or Part C due process procedures for families of children served under Part C of the IDEA. This

---

[57] Part C extends "The right of parents to use mediation in accordance with section 615, except that—(A) any reference in the section to a State educational agency shall be considered to be a reference to a State's lead agency established or designated under section 635(a)(10); (B) any reference in the section to a local educational agency shall be considered to be a reference to a local service provider or the State's lead agency under this part, as the case may be; and (C) any reference in the section to the provision of a free appropriate public education to children with disabilities shall be considered to be a reference to the provision of appropriate early intervention services to infants and toddlers with disabilities." (Part B: 20 U.S.C. §1415(e), P.L. 108-446 §615(e) and 34 C.F.R. §300.506 (2010). Part C: 20 U.S.C. §1439(a), P.L. 108-446 §639(a)(8)).

chapter will first discuss the due process complaint procedures developed for Part C and then will examine the differences between the IDEA Part B and Part C due process procedures.

Part C Due Process Procedures

The Part C due process complaint procedure begins with filing a due process complaint, which is in effect a request for a due process hearing, on matters relating to the identification, evaluation, or assessment of an infant or toddler with a disability, or the provision of appropriate early intervention services to the infant or toddler. Generally, unless the state's lead agency or the local service provider and the parent otherwise agree, the infant or toddler must continue to receive the appropriate early intervention services in the setting identified in his or her IFSP pending the outcome of the due process complaint procedures or of a court proceeding.[58]

A parent, early intervention service provider, or lead agency may file a due process complaint. The due process complaint must allege a violation that occurred not more than one year prior to the date that the complaint is received by the lead agency.[59] Each lead agency must ensure that, not later than 30 days after the receipt of a parent's due process complaint, the due process hearing is completed and a written decision mailed to each of the parties.[60] The due process hearing is conducted by an impartial hearing officer.[61] Any party aggrieved by the findings and decision issued pursuant to a due process complaint has the right to bring a civil action in state or federal court.[62]

---

[58] 20 U.S.C. §1439(b), P.L. 108-446 §639(b) and 34 C.F.R. §300.430 (e).

[59] There are two exceptions to this timeline. The timeline does not apply if (1) the parent was prevented from requesting a hearing due to specific misrepresentations by the local service provider that it had resolved the problem forming the basis of the due process complaint, or (2) the local service provider withheld information from the parent that was required to be provided to the parent. 20 U.S.C. §1415(b)(6), P.L. 108-446 §615(b)(6), and 34 C.F.R. §303.443 (2010).

[60] The only exception to this timeline is in cases where one of the parties requests and is granted an extension by the hearing officer. 34 C.F.R. §303.437.

[61] For information on conducting a due process hearing, for Part B see 20 U.S.C. §1415(f), P.L. 108-446 §615(f), for Part C see 34 C.F.R. §§303.435-438. For information on the required qualifications of the hearing officer, see 34 C.F.R. §303.435.

[62] For more detail, see the regulatory provisions at 34 C.F.R. §303.438 (2010).

Differences between the IDEA Part B and Part C Due Process Procedures

The Part B due process regulations contain additional steps and procedures that states which elect to use them must follow.[63] U.S. Department of Education officials suggest that the requirement that states that chose to implement Part B due process procedures for hearings involving children served under Part C abide by additional procedures, explains a large part of why many more states choose to adopt Part C due process procedures rather than adopt Part B due process procedures.[64]

Table 1. Due Process Procedures for Complaints Under Part C of the IDEA

States and Outlying Areas Using Part B Due Process Procedures			**States and Outlying Areas Using Part C Due Process Procedures**	
Alabama	Northern Marianas	Alaska	Kansas	Pennsylvania
District of	Ohio	American Samoa	Kentucky	Puerto Rico
Columbia	Oklahoma	Arizona	Louisiana	Rhode Island
Florida	Oregon	Arkansas	Massachusetts	South Carolina
Guam	South Dakota	California	Mississippi	Texas
Illinois	Tennessee	Colorado	Missouri	Utah
Maryland	Vermont	Connecticut	Montana	Virgin Islands
Maine		Delaware	New Hampshire	Virginia
Michigan		Georgia	New Jersey	Washington
Minnesota		Hawaii	New Mexico	West Virginia
Nebraska		Idaho	New York	Wisconsin
Nevada		Indiana	North Carolina	Wyoming
		Iowa	North Dakota	

Source: Table prepared by CRS. Information collected from Lead Agencies' 2015 Annual Performance Reports (FFY 2013) to the U.S. Department of Education Office of Special Education Programs (OSEP) by the national Center for Appropriate Dispute Resolution in Special Education (CADRE).

---

[63] For more information on the Part B due process procedures for children with disabilities ages 3 to 21 years old, see CRS Report R41833, *The Individuals with Disabilities Education Act (IDEA), Part B: Key Statutory and Regulatory Provisions*.

[64] 34 C.F.R. Part 303 (2010). Analysis of Comments and Changes: *States That Choose to Adopt the Part B Due Process Procedures under Section 615 of the Act* (§§303.440 through 303.447).

In 2013, 15 states, the District of Columbia, Guam, and the Northern Marianas Islands reported exercising the option to adopt the Part B due process procedures, while the remaining 35 states, Puerto Rico, American Samoa, and the U.S. Virgin Islands reported adopting the Part C due process procedures (see *Table 1* for a complete listing).

In some states that adopted the Part B due process procedures, the Part C lead agency is the SEA. In such states, the SEA administers both Parts B and C of the IDEA. In addition, in some states that use the Part B due process procedures, children receiving services under Part C of the act are also entitled under state law to some of the principal protections afforded to children under Part B, primarily the right to receive a free and appropriate public education (FAPE). These states provide parents with procedural protections under both Parts B and C of the IDEA.[65]

State Complaint Procedures[66]

The IDEA regulations require each state lead agency to adopt written procedures for resolving complaints that allege the lead agency, public agency, or early intervention services provider has violated a requirement of the Part C statute or regulations. In its analysis of comments and changes to the final Part B regulations, ED distinguishes between the due process complaint process and the state complaint process as follows:

> The due process complaint procedures and the State complaint procedures are separate and distinct. The State complaint procedures remain a viable alternative to the due process procedures for parents to resolve disputes with public agencies in a less formal and more cost effective manner.[67]

---

[65] 34 C.F.R. Part 303 (2010). Analysis of Comments and Changes: States That Choose to Adopt the Part B Due Process Procedures under Section 615 of the Act (§§303.440 through 303.447).

[66] 34 C.F.R. §303.432 through §303.334 (2010).

[67] 71 Fed. Reg. 46700 (August 14, 2006).

Unlike requests for mediation or for complaints filed under due process procedures, where only a parent, early intervention service provider, or a lead agency can file a complaint, a state complaint can be filed by any organization or individual, including those from another state. State complaint procedures must ensure that complaints will be resolved within 60 calendar days from the date the complaint is filed unless an extension is permitted.[68]

FUNDING, EXPENDITURE REQUIREMENTS, AND COMPLIANCE

The IDEA provides federal funding for early intervention programs for infants and toddlers with disabilities and developmental delays and imposes certain conditions for the receipt of federal funds. This section addresses (1) the structure and funding of the IDEA; (2) state formula allocations and expenditure requirements; and (3) the responsibilities of lead agencies, early intervention service providers, and parents regarding paying for early intervention services.

Structure and Funding of the IDEA

The IDEA consists of four parts. Part A contains general provisions, including the purposes of the act and definitions that apply to the entire act. Part B contains provisions relating to the education of school aged children (the grants-to-states program) and state grants program for preschool children with disabilities (Section 619).[69] Part C, the focus of this chapter,

---

[68] An extension of the 60-day time limit may be permitted only if exceptional circumstances exist with respect to a particular complaint or if the complainant and the lead agency, public agency, or early intervention services provider agree to extend the time to engage in mediation.

[69] For more information on funding for Part B of the IDEA, see CRS Report R41833, The Individuals with Disabilities Education Act (IDEA), Part B: Key Statutory and Regulatory Provisions.

authorizes state grants for programs serving infants and toddlers with disabilities. Finally, Part D contains the requirements for various national activities designed to improve the education of children with disabilities. *Table 2* shows the structure and funding of the IDEA. *Appendix A* provides a more detailed summary of each of the four parts.

Table 2. Structure and Funding of the IDEA (Funding in thousands of dollars)

IDEA Part	Description	FY2018 Funding	Percentage of Total IDEA Funding
Part A—General Provisions	Includes findings, purposes, and definitions	—	—
Part B—Assistance for Education of all Children with Disabilities	Contains provisions relating to the education of school aged children (the grants-to-states program) and state grants program for preschool children with disabilities (Section 619)	$12,658,968[a]	94.8%
Part C—Infants and Toddlers with Disabilities	Authorizes state grants for programs serving infants and toddlers with disabilities	$470,000	3.5%
Part D—National Activities to Improve Education of Children with Disabilities	Contains the requirements for various national activities	$222,133	1.7%
IDEA Total		$13,351,101	100%

Source: Table prepared by CRS. Funding amounts are from Department of Education budget tables for FY2018.

[a] Of this amount, $381.1 million, or 2.8% of the total IDEA FY2018 appropriation, was appropriated for the state grants program for preschool children with disabilities (Section 619).

While funding for Part B, Assistance for Education of all Children with Disabilities, is permanently authorized, the 2004 reauthorization of the IDEA authorized funding for Part C, Infants and Toddlers with Disabilities, and Part D, National Activities, through FY2010. These authorities were automatically extended for an additional fiscal year by the General

Education Provisions Act (GEPA).[70] Funding for Part C continues to be authorized through annual appropriations. In FY2017, $458.6 million was appropriated for Part C, representing 3.5% of total IDEA funding. *Appendix B* provides the amounts appropriated for Part C each year since the 2004 reauthorization and *Appendix C* displays funding levels for Part C in both actual and constant dollar amounts from the program's first year of funding in FY1987 through FY2017. Annual funding for each state for Part C programs is based upon each state's relative share of the general population birth through two. The IDEA is administered by the Office of Special Education Programs (OSEP) in the Office of Special Education and Rehabilitative Services (OSERS) in the Department of Education (ED).

State Formula Allocations

Of the funds appropriated for Part C of the IDEA, the Secretary may reserve no more than 1% of the appropriation for the outlying areas,[71] and must reserve 1.25% of the appropriation for tribes, tribal organizations, and consortia of those groups for the provision of early intervention services on reservations.[72] The remaining Part C funds are allocated to the 50 states, the District of Columbia, and Puerto Rico according to the ratio of infants and toddlers in each state to the number of infants and toddlers in all states. The minimum allotment for each state is either $500,000 or one-half of 1% of the total Part C funds allotted to the states, whichever is greater. If the appropriation for Part C is reduced to a level insufficient to pay the full amounts that all states are eligible to receive in a given year, the Secretary

---

[70] General Education Provisions Act (GEPA; 20 U.S.C. §1226a). For more information see CRS Report R41119, *General Education Provisions Act (GEPA): Overview and Issues*.

[71] 20 U.S.C. §1411(b)(1), P.L. 108-446 §616(b)(1). The outlying areas are defined in §602(22) as the "United States Virgin Islands, Guam, American Samoa, and the Commonwealth of the Northern Mariana Islands." Part C §643(2) further states "The provisions of Public Law 95–134, permitting the consolidation of grants to the outlying areas, shall not apply to funds those areas receive under this part."

[72] Section 643(b)(1) reserves 1.25% of the Part C appropriation for the Department of the Interior for the "coordination of assistance in the provision of early intervention services by the States to infants and toddlers with disabilities and their families on reservations served by elementary schools and secondary schools for Indian children operated or funded by the Department of the Interior."

must ratably reduce the states' payments, meaning the reduction will be proportionately reflected in the allotment for each state.[73]

State Expenditure Requirements

Part C does not require states to create new early intervention systems for children with disabilities under three years of age; instead, it requires the coordination of existing early intervention services into one accessible system. States use IDEA funds to coordinate these services through state interagency agreements, contracts, and cooperative arrangements. Therefore, Part C grants finance primarily administrative functions, and do not directly provide services.

The IDEA state expenditure requirements are aimed at increasing overall early intervention spending, rather than substituting federal funds for early intervention spending at the state and local levels. Supplement, not supplant (SNS) requirements generally prohibit a state or lead agency from using IDEA grants to provide services, purchase equipment, and so forth, that state, local, or other federal funds currently provide or purchase or, in the absence of the IDEA funds, that those other funds would have provided or would have purchased. Both states and lead agencies must use IDEA funds to supplement state, local, and other federal funds and not to supplant them.[74]

Who Pays for Early Intervention Services?

Depending on the state's policies, parents of infants and toddlers with disabilities may have to pay for certain early intervention services. Parents may be charged a sliding-scale fee for some services, based on what they earn. However, early intervention services cannot be denied to a child simply

[73] If additional funds become available for making payments for a fiscal year in which payments to states were ratably reduced, the allotments that were reduced must be increased on the same basis the allotments were reduced. §643(c)(3).

[74] 20 U.S.C. §1437(b)(5)(B), P.L. 108-446 §637(b)(5)(B).

because his or her family is not able to pay for services, and Part C of the IDEA requires the following services to be provided at no cost to families: Child Find services; evaluations and assessments; the development and review of the IFSP; and service coordination.

A description of the state's payment system must be made available in writing and given to the parents of participating children at the beginning of the early intervention process. Some early intervention services may be covered by parents' health insurance, by Medicaid, or by the Indian Health Service. The Part C system may ask parents for their permission to access their public or private insurance in order to pay for their child's early intervention services. In most cases, the early intervention system may not use a family's health care insurance (private or public) without their express, written consent. If the family denies consent, the early intervention system may not limit or refuse to provide services for them or their child.

APPENDIX A. STRUCTURE OF THE IDEA

Part A: General Provisions

Part A includes congressional findings pertinent to the act, the purposes of the act, and definitions. These definitions include, among others, definitions of child with a disability, specific learning disability, free appropriate public education, core academic subjects, highly qualified, individualized education program, local educational agency, related services, special education, supplementary aids and services, transition services, and excess costs.

Part B: Assistance for Education of All Children with Disabilities

Part B authorizes federal funding for the education of children with disabilities and requires, as a condition for the receipt of such funds, the provision of a free appropriate public education (FAPE) to children with disabilities between the ages of 3 and 21. Provisions in Part B require that school districts must identify, locate, and evaluate all children with disabilities, regardless of the severity of their disability, to determine which children are eligible for special education and related services. Further, they require that each child receiving services has an Individualized Education Program (IEP), created by an IEP team, delineating the specific special education and related services to be provided to meet his or her needs. The statute also contains procedural safeguards, which are provisions to protect the rights of parents and children with disabilities to ensure the provision of FAPE.

Section 619 of IDEA Part B authorizes grants to states for preschool programs serving children with disabilities ages three to five. Since Part B grants to states are used to serve children with disabilities as young as three years of age (as well as school-age children), Section 619 is not so much a separate program as it is supplementary funding for services to this age group. In general, the provisions, requirements, and guarantees under the grants to states program that apply to school-age children with disabilities also apply to children in this age group. As a result, Section 619 is a relatively brief section of the law and deals primarily with the state and substate funding formulas for the grants and state-level activities.

Part C: Infants and Toddlers with Disabilities

The general purpose of Part C is to aid each state in creating and maintaining "a statewide, comprehensive, coordinated, multidisciplinary, interagency system that provides early intervention services for infants and toddlers with disabilities and their families."[75] The provisions in Part C require that services focus on children from birth through age two who are experiencing or have a high probability of experiencing "developmental delay" (as defined by the state) with respect to physical, mental, or other

[75] 20 U.S.C. §1431(b)(1), P.L. 108-446 §631(b)(1).

capacities, and on their families.[76] Services are detailed for each child and his or her family in an Individualized Family Service Plan (IFSP). Services are to be provided, to the maximum extent feasible, in "natural environments," including the home, with other infants and toddlers who are not disabled. Under the provisions of Part C, states are required to identify a state lead agency, which might be the state educational agency (SEA) but could be other state agencies, to coordinate the program.

Part D: National Activities to Improve Education of Children with Disabilities[77]

Part D authorizes competitive grants to improve the education of children with disabilities in three areas: (1) state personnel development (Subpart 1); (2) personnel preparation, technical assistance, model demonstration projects, and dissemination of information (Subpart 2); and (3) support to improve results for children (Subpart 3).

- Under Subpart 1, state personnel development grants are authorized. These grants assist SEAs "in reforming and improving their systems for personnel preparation and professional development in early intervention, educational, and transitions services."[78]
- Under Subpart 2, a competitive grants program is authorized through which grants are made to entities such as SEAs, LEAs, institutions of higher education (IHEs), and nonprofit organizations for personnel development to help ensure that there are adequate numbers of personnel with skills and knowledge needed to help

---

[76] Under certain circumstances, children with disabilities age three and over may continue to receive Part C early intervention services until they are eligible to enter kindergarten; 20 U.S.C. §14345(c), P.L. 108-446 §635(c).

[77] In addition to the statutory provisions in Part D, see the following for more information on these activities: U.S. Department of Education, *Fiscal Year 2019, Budget Summary*, pp. 19-21; and U.S. Department of Education, *Guide to U.S. Department of Education Programs,2012*, pp. 239-247.

[78] 20 U.S.C. §1451(a), P.L. 108-446 §651(a).

children with disabilities succeed, for technical assistance and dissemination of material based on knowledge gained through research and practice, and for studies and evaluations.

- Under Subpart 3, a competitive grants program is authorized through which grants are made to nonprofit organizations for parent training and information centers, which provide parents of children with disabilities with needed training and information to work with professionals in meeting the early intervention and special education needs of their children.[79] Also, under Subpart 3, competitive grants are authorized for entities such as SEAs, LEAs, IHEs, and nonprofit organizations to support research, development, and other activities that promote the use of technology in providing special education and early intervention services.[80]

APPENDIX B. IDEA, PART C APPROPRIATIONS

Table B-1. IDEA, Part C Grants to States: Appropriations from FY2004 to FY2018

Fiscal Year	Appropriation (in millions)
2004	$444.4
2005	$440.8
2006	$436.4
2007	$436.4
2008	$435.7
2009	$439.4
2010	$439.4
2011	$438.6
2012	$442.7
2013	$419.7

[79] 20 U.S.C. §1471, §1472, and §1473, P.L. 108-446 §671, §672, and §673.
[80] 20 U.S.C. §1474, P.L. 108-446 §674.

Fiscal Year	Appropriation (in millions)
2014	$438.5
2015	$438.6
2016	$458.6
2017	$458.6
2018	$470.0

Source: Table created by CRS based on FY2004 to FY2018 appropriation data from the U.S. Department of Education.

Note: FY2013 amount reflects sequestration.

APPENDIX C. THE FIRST 30 YEARS OF PART C FUNDING

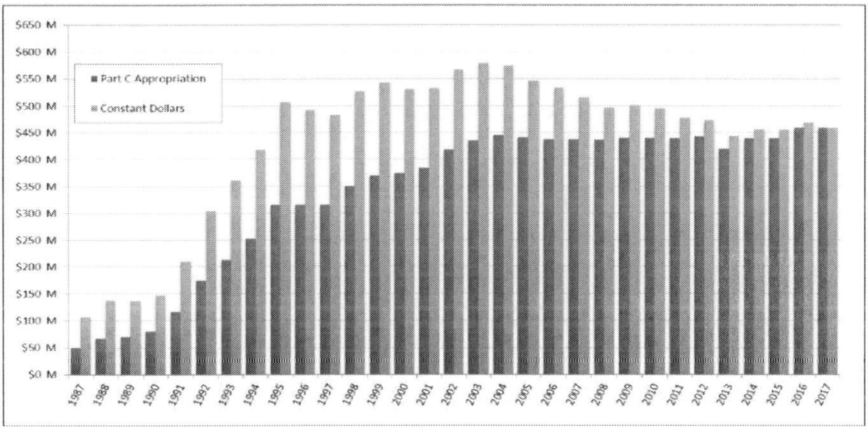

Source: Figure prepared by CRS. Funding amounts are from U.S. Department of Education budget tables.

Notes: Constant dollar amounts show inflation-adjusted funding amounts calculated using the Consumer Price Index–All Urban Consumers (CPI-U).

The funding amount for FY2009 only displays regular appropriations; additional IDEA funding provided by the American Recovery and Reinvestment Act (ARRA) is not displayed.

Figure C-1. Part C, Infants and Families Program Funding, FY1987-FY2017. (Funding in millions, shown in actual and constant FY2017 dollar amounts)

APPENDIX D. COMMONLY USED ACRONYMS

APPE	Average Per Pupil Expenditure
APR	Annual Performance Report
ED	U.S. Department of Education
EI	Early Intervention
EIS	Early Intervention Services
ESEA	Elementary and Secondary Education Act
FAPE	Free Appropriate Public Education
IDEA	Individuals with Disabilities Education Act
IEP	Individualized Education Program
IFSP	Individualized Family Services Plan
LEA	Local Educational Agency
MOE	Maintenance of Effort
SEA	State Education Agency
SNS	Supplement, Not Supplant
SPP	State Performance Plan

In: Individuals with Disabilities
Editor: Aston Delgado

ISBN: 978-1-53615-030-8

Chapter 4

STUDENTS WITH DISABILITIES: ADDITIONAL INFORMATION FROM EDUCATION COULD HELP STATES PROVIDE PRE-EMPLOYMENT TRANSITION SERVICES*

United States Government Accountability Office

ABBREVIATIONS

CSAVR	Council of State Administrators of Vocational Rehabilitation
Education	U.S. Department of Education
IDEA	Individuals with Disabilities Education Act
IEP	individualized education program
NCSAB	National Council of State Agencies for the Blind
NTACT	National Technical Assistance Center

* This is an edited, reformatted and augmented version of United States Government Accountability Office; Report to the Ranking Member, Committee on Health, Education, Labor, and Pensions, U.S. Senate, Publication No. GAO-18-502, dated September 2018.

	on Transition
Rehabilitation Act	Rehabilitation Act of 1973
RSA	Rehabilitation Services Administration
VR	vocational rehabilitation
WIOA	Workforce Innovation and Opportunity Act
WINTAC	Workforce Innovation Technical Assistance Center

Why GAO Did This Study

WIOA requires states to reserve at least 15 percent of their total State Vocational Rehabilitation Services program funds to provide pre-employment transition services to help students with disabilities transition from school to work. GAO was asked to review how states were implementing these services.

This chapter examines (1) steps states reported taking to implement pre-employment transition services, and (2) implementation challenges states reported and how Education has addressed them. GAO reviewed documents and funding data from Education, and federal laws and regulations; surveyed all 79 state VR agencies (74 responded); held discussion groups with representatives of 29 state VR agencies; and interviewed officials from Education and three states (Idaho, Illinois, and Maryland) GAO selected for variety in size and type of agencies, among other factors.

What GAO Recommends

GAO is recommending that Education (1) establish timeframes for providing additional information on allowable expenditures, (2) take additional steps to assist states that have not updated and finalized their interagency agreements, and (3) develop a written plan with specific timeframes and activities for identifying and disseminating best practices.

Education agreed with the first recommendation and disagreed with the other two. GAO revised the second recommendation and maintains that specific information is needed for the third, as discussed in the report.

WHAT GAO FOUND

Of the 74 state vocational rehabilitation (VR) agencies that responded to GAO's survey, most reported expanding services to help students with disabilities transition from school to work as required under the Workforce Innovation and Opportunity Act (WIOA), enacted in July 2014. Most state agencies reported serving more students and providing work-based learning experiences and other activities, referred to as pre-employment transition services (see Figure).

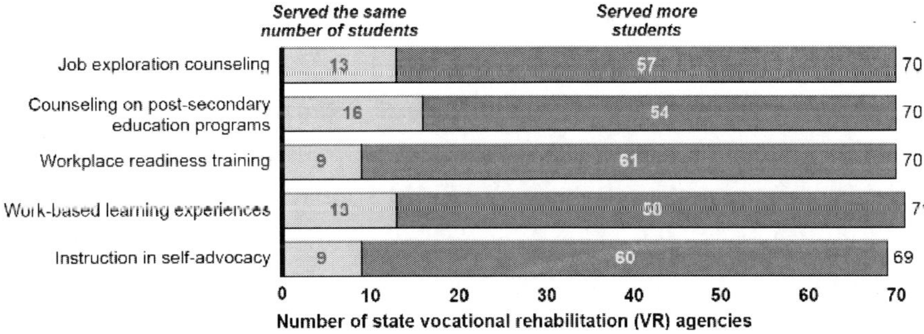

Source: GAO survey of State VR agencies. | GAO-18-502.

Note: There were 74 respondents. Totals do not sum to 74 because for each service one respondent reported decreases in the number of students served and the remainder either did not answer the question or responded "don't know."

Number of Agencies That Reported Serving More Students Since July 2014. State VR agencies reported two key challenges with implementing pre-employment transition services for students as required by WIOA.

Spending Reserved Funds

States reported spending about $357 million out of the $465 million reserved for these services in fiscal year 2016. Education officials said that states had difficulty determining what expenditures were allowable, and some state officials said they would like more detailed information from Education. Education officials said they plan to clarify guidance but have no timeframe for providing further information, which would help states to better plan their use of reserved funds.

Finalizing Interagency Agreements

Fewer than half the state VR agencies that responded to GAO's survey (34 of 74) reported updating their interagency agreement with their state's educational agency. Interagency agreements can help promote collaboration by, for example, establishing roles and responsibilities of each agency. Although Education offers technical assistance on interagency agreements, without increased efforts to raise awareness about the importance of these agreements and provide assistance to states where needed, Education may miss opportunities to help state VR and educational agencies efficiently and effectively coordinate services.

In addition, WIOA requires Education to highlight best state practices, and most VR agencies responding to GAO's survey (63 of 74) reported this would be useful. Education does not have a written plan or timeframe for identifying and disseminating best practices. As a result, Education may miss opportunities to help more students with disabilities successfully transition from school to work.

September 6, 2018
The Honorable Patty Murray
Ranking Member
Committee on Health, Education, Labor, and Pensions
United States Senate

Dear Senator Murray:

The transition from high school to postsecondary education or the workforce can be a challenging time for students, and particularly for those with disabilities who may need additional services or guidance to achieve their goals. We have reported that students with disabilities are less likely than their peers to transition successfully.[1] In addition, people with disabilities have historically experienced higher unemployment and poverty rates than those without disabilities.[2] Students with disabilities who do not successfully transition from school to the workforce may face a lifetime of reliance on public assistance, potentially leading to substantial costs to the government and society. While states provide transition services through special education in schools and to some students who apply and are determined eligible for the State Vocational Rehabilitation Services program, the Workforce Innovation and Opportunity Act (WIOA) amended the Rehabilitation Act of 1973 (Rehabilitation Act) in 2014 to require states to additionally provide a defined set of activities called pre-employment transition services.[3] These services are to be provided both to students who are eligible for the program as well as to those who are potentially eligible, greatly expanding the number of students who can be served. Pre-employment transition services are offered as an early start on job exploration and are designed to help these students identify their career interests. Specifically, states are required to offer job exploration counseling and work-based learning experiences, which may include internships, exposures to local employment, and other activities.

---

[1] GAO, *Students with Disabilities: Better Federal Coordination Could Lessen Challenges in the Transition from High School*, GAO-12-594 (Washington, D.C.; July 12, 2012).

[2] U.S. Department of Labor, Bureau of Labor Statistics, *Labor Force Statistics from the Current Population Survey*, (Washington, D.C.: Data extracted on June 11, 2018); and U.S. Department of Commerce, Economics and Statistics Administration, U.S. Census Bureau, *Income and Poverty in the United States: 2016, Current Population Reports,* P60- 259 (Washington, D.C.: September 2017).

[3] Pub. L. No. 113-128, § 422, 128 Stat. 1425, 1657 (2014) (codified at 29 U.S.C. § 733). The State Vocational Rehabilitation Services program provides services that, among other things, help individuals, including students with disabilities obtain employment, including counseling and training. To be eligible, an individual must be an "individual with a disability," which means that the individual has a physical or mental impairment which constitutes or results in a substantial impediment to employment and can benefit in terms of an employment outcome from vocational rehabilitation services.

In fiscal year 2017, the Department of Education (Education) awarded about $3.1 billion in grants to states for the State Vocational Rehabilitation Services program. WIOA requires states to reserve at least 15 percent of their vocational rehabilitation (VR) grants to provide preemployment transition services to all eligible or potentially eligible students with disabilities who need them.[4] That reserve amounted to about $468 million across all states in fiscal year 2017.

You asked us to provide information on how states are implementing pre-employment transition services. This chapter examines (1) the steps states have reported taking to implement pre-employment transition services, and (2) the implementation challenges, if any, states have reported facing, and how Education has addressed them.

To obtain information on both of these objectives, we used the following methodologies. We reviewed Education's guidance and technical assistance documents as well as federal laws and regulations.[5] We reviewed expenditure data reported by state VR agencies to Education for fiscal years 2015 and 2016, the most recent full years of data available, and determined they were reliable for the purposes of this review by interviewing Education officials about the data's quality and by electronically testing the data for any obvious errors. We administered a web-based survey to all 79 state VR agencies from October through December 2017, with 74 agencies (94 percent) responding.[6] We conducted interviews with state VR and educational officials in Idaho, Illinois, and Maryland. We selected these states based on variety in the size of the special education population, state

---

[4] The statutory requirements governing the State Vocational Rehabilitation Services program, including those related to the provision of pre-employment transition services, are found in the Rehabilitation Act of 1973 (Rehabilitation Act), as amended by Title IV of the Workforce Innovation and Opportunity Act (WIOA). However, because this report focuses on certain requirements added to the Rehabilitation Act by WIOA, for ease of reference we refer to these provisions as WIOA requirements.

[5] We did not assess states' compliance with WIOA requirements; rather, this report conveys information that states reported to us about steps they have taken and the challenges they faced in implementing pre-employment transition services.

[6] In this report, the term *state VR agencies* refers to agencies in the 50 states, the District of Columbia, and the territories of American Samoa, Guam, Northern Marianas, Puerto Rico, and the Virgin Islands. Twenty-three states have two VR agencies: one dedicated to serving the blind and visually impaired and another designed to serve all other individuals with disabilities. Twenty-seven states, the District of Columbia, and 5 territories have one combined VR agency.

agency organization, and whether the state had a separate agency for serving individuals who are blind or visually impaired. The information from these interviews is not generalizable. We interviewed representatives of other relevant organizations, including the Council of State Administrators of Vocational Rehabilitation (CSAVR) and the National Council of State Agencies for the Blind. In addition, we interviewed officials from Education's Office of Special Education and Rehabilitation Services, Rehabilitation Services Administration, Office of Special Education Programs, and the Workforce Innovation Technical Assistance Center and National Technical Assistance Center on Transition—two technical assistance centers funded by Education. We also convened three discussion groups with state VR agency directors or their designated representatives, with a total of 39 participants from 29 separate agencies (10 to 12 agencies represented per discussion group). We invited all state VR agencies to participate through our survey and through the conference organizer (CSAVR). To assess how Education addressed challenges reported by state VR agencies, we compared actions taken by Education to standards for internal control in the federal government. For further details on our objectives, scope, and methodology, see appendix I.

We conducted this performance audit from February 2017 to September 2018 in accordance with generally accepted government auditing standards. Those standards require that we plan and perform the audit to obtain sufficient, appropriate evidence to provide a reasonable basis for our findings and conclusions based on our audit objectives. We believe that the evidence obtained provides a reasonable basis for our findings and conclusions based on our audit objectives.

BACKGROUND

The Rehabilitation Act of 1973 (Rehabilitation Act), as amended by WIOA, authorizes a number of grant programs to support employment and independent living for persons with disabilities, including the State

Vocational Rehabilitation Services program.[7] This program is the primary federal government effort to help individuals with disabilities prepare for and obtain employment. An individual who is deemed eligible works with state VR agency staff to prepare an individualized plan for employment, which describes the employment goal and the specific services needed to achieve that goal. Education's Rehabilitation Services Administration (RSA) awards funds to state VR agencies through the program to help individuals with disabilities engage in gainful employment. States must provide a 21.3 percent nonfederal match of these funds. In fiscal year 2016, total program funds for VR—including state match funds—were $3.81 billion.

States, territories, and the District of Columbia generally designate a single agency to administer the program, although, depending on state law, states may designate more than one agency. Twenty-three states have two separate agencies, one that exclusively serves blind and visually impaired individuals (known as agencies for the blind) and another that serves individuals who are not blind or visually impaired (known as general agencies). Twenty-seven states, the District of Columbia, and the five territories have a single combined agency that serves both blind and visually impaired individuals and individuals with other types of impairments (known as combined agencies). In total, there are 79 state VR agencies.

Pre-Employment Transition Services

In 2014, WIOA amended the Rehabilitation Act to require state VR agencies to provide students with disabilities with pre-employment transition services. According to information Education provided with its regulations, WIOA emphasized the provision of services to students with disabilities to ensure that they have meaningful opportunities to receive training and other supports and services they need to achieve employment outcomes.

---

[7] Rehabilitation Act of 1973, Pub. L. No. 93-112, 87 Stat. 355 (codified as amended at 29 U.S.C. §§ 701-796l).

Table 1. Pre-employment Transition Services Activities Required by the Workforce Innovation and Opportunity Act (WIOA) for Students with Disabilities, and Examples of Each Activity

Activity	Description
Job exploration counseling	Discussing local labor market information, including in-demand industry sectors and occupations, as well as nontraditional employment and career pathways of interest to the students, as well as administering vocational interest inventories.
Work-based learning experiences	Coordinating such experiences as a school-based program of job training and informational interviews to research employers; work-site tours to learn about necessary job skills, job shadowing, or mentoring opportunities in the community; internships, apprenticeships, short-term employment, and fellowships (paid or unpaid), or on-the-job trainings located in the community.
Post-secondary activity counseling	Providing information on course offerings, career options, and the types of academic and occupational training needed to succeed in the workplace, and postsecondary opportunities associated with career fields or pathways.
Workplace readiness training	Helping students with disabilities develop social skills and independent living skills (financial literacy and travel skills); job-seeking skills; and an understanding of employer expectations for punctuality and performance, as well as other "soft" skills necessary for employment.
Self-advocacy	Teaching students about their rights and responsibilities, including how to request accommodations or services and supports and communicate their thoughts, concerns, and needs in the area of education or employment interests.

Source: WIOA and the U.S. Department of Education. | GAO-18-502.

WIOA requires states to make pre-employment transition services available statewide to all students with disabilities in need of such services, who are eligible or potentially eligible, regardless of whether a student has submitted an application for services from a state VR agency.[8] In this

[8] See 29 U.S.C. §§ 705(37) and 733(a). WIOA requires each state to prepare a Unified or Combined State Plan once every 4 years that describes the goals, services, and objectives of its workforce development system. RSA approves the VR services portion of the State Plan, which must include information on formal interagency agreements between the state VR and educational agency that provides for, among other things, procedures for identifying students with disabilities who need pre-employment transition services. Education and the U.S. Department of Labor review and approve each state's Unified or Combined State Plan.

context, students with disabilities include those with an individualized education program (IEP) for special education services through the school system, those receiving an accommodation for their disability, and others.[9] In information provided with the regulations, Education stated that state VR agencies should work closely with school systems and others to identify these students. WIOA requires each state to reserve at least 15 percent of a state's VR allotment for a fiscal year for pre-employment transition services for students with disabilities.[10] If a state cannot use or match all of its VR funding, it relinquishes funds to the federal government and the state's total award amount is then reduced.[11] However, the state must still reserve 15 percent of what it did not relinquish for the provision of preemployment transition services.

WIOA established required activities under pre-employment transition services that states must make available to students with disabilities.

Education has provided states with additional information about each of the activities (see Table 1).

After making the required pre-employment transition services available, if a state has funding remaining, WIOA lists nine other "authorized" activities that a state may implement. For example, in providing the

---

[9] The Individuals with Disabilities Education Act (IDEA) requires that school districts or state educational agencies provide an IEP for all students determined eligible for special education services. The IEP is developed at a meeting by a team that includes, among others, school officials, other educational professionals, and parents. IEP team meetings may also include a representative of any participating agency that is likely to be responsible for providing or paying for transition services. The IEP includes a student's academic performance, academic and functional goals, special education and related services, and other supports to enable advancement toward these goals. See 20 U.S.C. §§ 1412(a)(4) and 1414(d).

[10] The formula for VR state grant allotments incorporates each state's population, average per capita income, and the VR allotment in 1978. WIOA did not provide new funding to states for providing pre-employment transition services; rather, states provide preemployment transition services from their VR allotment.

[11] If at the end of the fiscal year a state has any unobligated funds remaining from its VR grant awarded in that fiscal year, and for which the state has been able to provide a nonfederal match, those funds can be carried forward into the subsequent fiscal year, including funds reserved for pre-employment transition services. States then have up to one year to obligate and expend the funds that were carried forward.

authorized activities, states may, among other things, provide training to local VR and educational service providers; coordinate transition services with local educational agencies; and disseminate information about innovative, effective, and efficient approaches to achieve the goals (see appendix II for a full listing of authorized activities). Education's guidance indicates that such authorized activities should improve the transition of students with disabilities from school to postsecondary education or an employment outcome and support the arrangement or provision of the required activities.

WIOA also requires local offices of state VR agencies to conduct coordination responsibilities, which includes coordinating with state and local educational agencies to ensure the provision of pre-employment transition services. These can be conducted concurrently with the "required" activities, and states can use the reserved funds for them. Examples of coordination responsibilities that local offices of state VR agencies must undertake are attending meetings, when invited, about IEPs; and working with the local public workforce system and employers to develop work opportunities for students with disabilities.

In support of this coordination and in recognition that VR and educational agencies both offer transition services to students, WIOA requires that VR agencies establish or update their interagency agreements with states educational agencies.[12] Interagency agreements between the state VR and educational agencies are intended to describe the steps each agency will take to implement pre-employment transition services and determine the roles and responsibilities of each agency, including financial responsibilities and procedures for identifying students in need of preemployment transition services.[13]

---

[12] Under the Individuals with Disabilities Education Act (IDEA), students with disabilities who may receive pre-employment transition services may also be eligible for transition services in schools as a part of special education. IDEA requires that, beginning no later than the student's first IEP that is in effect when the student turns 16 (or younger if determined appropriate by the IEP team), a student's IEP must include measurable postsecondary goals and the transition services needed to assist the student in reaching those goals. In many cases, the same activities can be considered pre-employment transition services, VR transition services, or IDEA transition services, according to Education.

[13] See 34 C.F.R. § 361.22(b).

Federal Guidance, Assistance, and Monitoring

Following the passage of WIOA, Education, through its Rehabilitation Services Administration (RSA), issued regulations and guidance to implement pre-employment transition services requirements (see Figure 1).

Education also provided technical assistance to state VR agencies through webinars, conference calls, and presentations at conferences. For example, Education presented information to state officials in a series of webinars about the new programmatic and financial processes and procedures related to pre-employment transition services just after the final regulations were issued in 2016. In addition, Education funded technical assistance centers to help state VR agencies and their partners answer questions and provide training about WIOA. Two of these centers are the Workforce Innovation Technical Assistance Center (WINTAC) and the National Technical Assistance Center on Transition (NTACT).[14] Each center focuses its efforts on a specific set of issues: WINTAC on helping state VR agencies implement WIOA requirements, including preemployment transition services; and NTACT on helping state VR and educational agencies improve outcomes for students receiving transition services.

RSA is to conduct periodic monitoring visits to assess state VR agencies' implementation of the VR program, including pre-employment transition services.[15] RSA is to monitor states for compliance with the administrative, financial, and performance requirements of the program, as well as identify technical assistance needs at individual state VR agencies.

---

[14] In addition to WINTAC and NTACT, Education funds another five technical assistance centers to provide help to state VR agencies in using their program to improve services to help maximize the employment of individuals with disabilities, and enhance their independence and integration into the community and the competitive labor market. WINTAC and NTACT, however, are the centers that provide the principal source of assistance regarding pre-employment transition services, according to Education officials.

[15] During the monitoring visits, RSA also assesses the Supported Employment Services program, which makes grants to states to provide time-limited supported employment services for individuals (both youth and adults) with the most significant disabilities, with the goal of supporting competitive integrated employment.

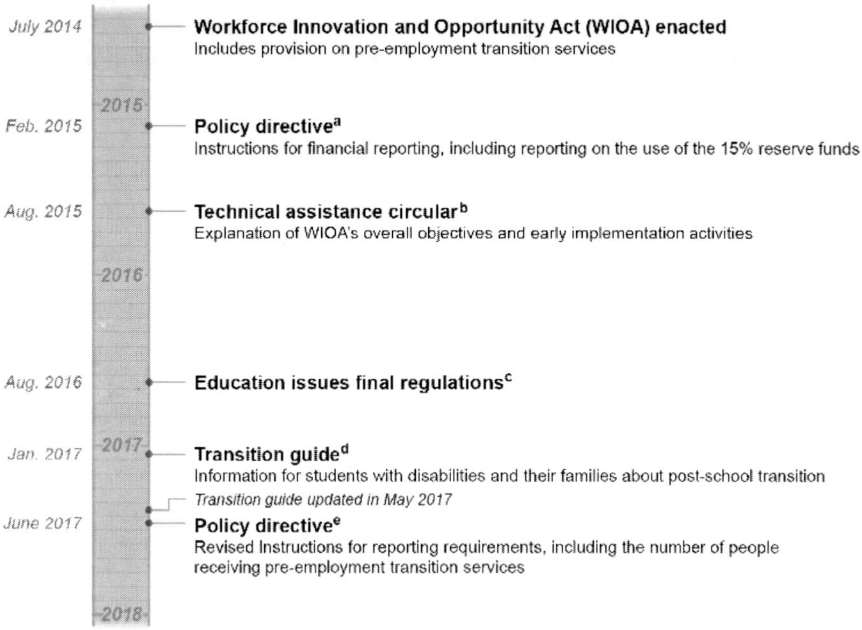

Source: GAO presentation of U.S. Department of Education information. | GAO-18-502.

[a]Education, Policy Directive: Revisions to PD-12-06, instructions for completing the Federal Financial Report (SF-425) for the State Vocational Rehabilitation Services program, RSA-PD-15-05, Feb. 5, 2015.

[b]Education, Technical Assistance Circular: Vision for the State Vocational Rehabilitation Services Program as a Partner in the Workforce Development System under the Workforce Innovation and Opportunity Act, RSA-TAC-15-02, Aug. 17, 2015.

[c]Education, State Vocational Rehabilitation Services Program; State Supported Employment Services Program; Limitation on Use of Subminimum Wage, 81 Fed. Reg. 55,630, (Aug. 19, 2016) (codified at 34 C.F.R. pts. 361, 363, and 397).

[d]Education, A Transition Guide to Postsecondary Education and Employment for Students and Youth with Disabilities, January 2017, and revised May 2017.

[e]Education, Policy Directive: Revision of Policy Directive 16-04 Instructions for the Completion of the Case Service Report Manual (RSA-911) for the State Vocational Rehabilitation Services Program and the State Supported Employment Services Program, RSA-PD-16-04, June 14, 2017.

Figure 1. Timeline of Key Guidance and Federal Regulations by Education Related to Pre-Employment Transition Services for Students with Disabilities After Enactment of the Workforce Innovation and Opportunity Act.

According to Education officials, RSA plans to follow a 5-year monitoring cycle that began in fiscal year 2017 and will generally include monitoring visits to 10 states per year through fiscal year 2021. In fiscal year 2017, Education visited 14 VR agencies in 10 states, and in fiscal year 2018, Education plans to visit 15 VR agencies in 12 states.

Most States Reported Expanding Their Transition Services to Students and Developing Their Administrative Capacity to Provide These Services

Most State Vocational Rehabilitation Agencies Reported Expanding Their Services for Students with Disabilities

Most state VR agencies that responded to our survey reported expanding services for students with disabilities since WIOA's enactment in July 2014 by either serving more students through pre-employment transition services or by initiating new or additional services. Most state VR agencies that responded to our survey reported that they provided the five required activities to more students with disabilities since WIOA's enactment (see Figure 2).[16]

State VR agencies indicated in their survey responses that they had previously provided and continue to provide transition services to students who apply and are eligible for the VR program, and many of the activities were not entirely new to state VR agencies. Most agencies that responded to our survey reported providing each of the required activities to students with disabilities before the enactment of WIOA, while fewer reported initiating these services since enactment (see Figure 3).

---

[16] According to Education officials, complete and reliable service provision data reported to Education were not available for the time of our review because Education just recently began collecting these data from states.

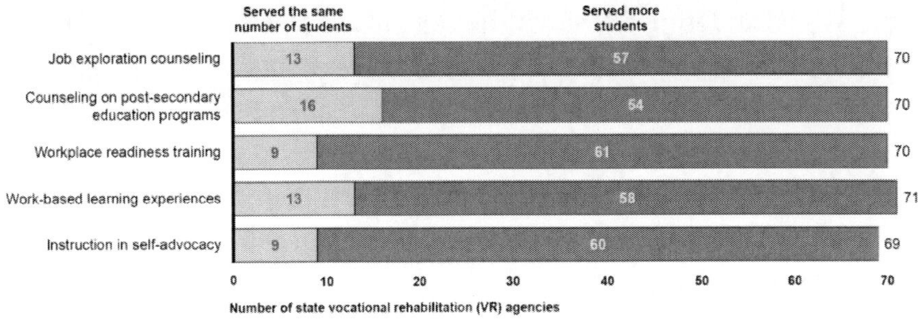

Source: GAO survey of state VR agencies. | GAO-18-502.

WIOA=Workforce Innovation and Opportunity Act.

Note: In instances in which the totals do not sum to 74, the remainder either responded "don't know," "decreased," or did not answer the question. One agency that reported decreases in the number of students being provided an activity also reported that it raised the minimum age for students to receive services.

Figure 2. Number of State Vocational Rehabilitation (VR) Agencies that Reported Increasing the Number of Students with Disabilities Receiving Services Since the Enactment of WIOA.

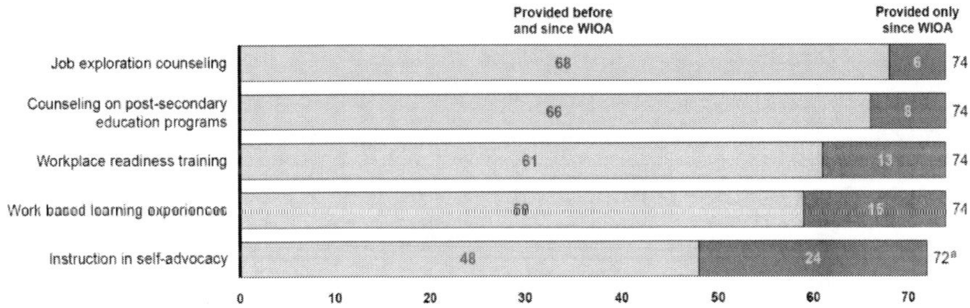

Source: GAO survey of state VR agencies. | GAO-18-502.

WIOA=Workforce Innovation and Opportunity Act.

[a]Two GAO survey respondents reported that they did not provide this service.

Figure 3. State Vocational Rehabilitation (VR) Agencies that Reported Providing the Five Required Pre-Employment Transition Services Activities for Students with Disabilities Before and Since the Enactment of WIOA.

Of the five required activities, instruction in self-advocacy saw the biggest expansion during this time. In information provided with the regulations, Education described instruction in self-advocacy as, for example, classroom lessons in which students learn about their rights, responsibilities, and how to request accommodations or services and supports needed during transition. In written comments on our survey, 10 state VR agencies reported partnering with other organizations, such as universities or centers for independent living, to provide instruction in self-advocacy. One agency reported on our survey that it offers peer mentoring as an additional component of self-advocacy services, and another reported providing self-advocacy and mentoring for deaf-blind students by deaf-blind adults. In October 2016, based on views of an expert panel that we convened on autism spectrum disorders and transitioning youth, we reported that it is critically important that all transitioning youth, regardless of their level of disability, be given the opportunity to state their own preferences to the extent of their capabilities to reach their maximum independence.[17]

State VR agencies reported developing additional programming as a result of WIOA's enactment, including expanding programs for more students, adding new opportunities and experiences, and creating new partnerships. Officials from all four of the state VR agencies we interviewed said they had programs in place prior to WIOA that offered activities similar to pre-employment transition services, but they have since expanded these services or created additional programs for students with disabilities. For example, an official we interviewed from the Idaho Division of Vocational Rehabilitation said the agency had previously worked to enroll students in the VR program prior to graduation, but has since begun developing new programming and instruction aimed at serving larger groups and providing other services, such as a paid work experience. An official from Maryland's Division of Rehabilitation Services said many of the services they previously offered were during school hours, and students had limited access to these services if they wanted to stay in class. The agency has since added services after school and during the summer, such as opportunities for students to meet with employers, according to Maryland officials. Officials from the Illinois Department of Human Services, Division of Rehabilitation Services, said that while the agency had previously provided work-based learning experiences, it has

---

[17] GAO, *Youth with Autism: Roundtable Views of Services Needed During the Transition into Adulthood,* GAO-17-109 (Washington, D.C.: October 18, 2016).

since expanded the number of spots available for students in an existing program and created a new work-based learning program that is a collaboration between school districts, a community rehabilitation partner, and businesses.

Providing new services with specific requirements to an expanded population has been a significant change, according to officials in one of the state VR agencies we interviewed and in all three of our discussion groups. For example, officials from Maryland's Division of Rehabilitation Services said that, while they provided all five required activities before WIOA, they now provide the activities to a younger population and make the activities available statewide. State VR officials in all three of our discussion groups said that providing pre-employment transition services allows them to provide these services to more students with disabilities or at an earlier age, which will likely have positive effects on students' transition from school to work. For example, officials in one discussion group noted that the provision of pre-employment transition services is increasing awareness, enhancing services, and increasing the likelihood that VR program outcomes will improve. In another discussion group, officials said their agencies had already seen benefits from preemployment transition services and the services have raised students' expectations for the types of jobs they might obtain.

While 32 of the state VR agencies responding to our survey reported that they had identified all potentially eligible students, another 37 reported that they were currently in the process of identifying these students.[18] State VR officials in all three of our discussion groups and who we interviewed in two of four state VR agencies said they have had challenges finding the population eligible for services. In written comments on our survey, one agency reported that while statewide information on students was not readily available, officials worked with the state educational agency to identify potentially eligible students, including more than 137,000 students with an IEP and an estimated 13,000 additional students that do not have an IEP.

[18] Four state VR agencies responded to our survey that they had not yet identified all students and one responded "don't know."

We previously reported on the difficulties state VR officials faced in obtaining data they could use to identify other youth with disabilities.[19]

Compared to combined and general agencies, more agencies for the blind reported in our survey that they did not provide the five required activities to more students with disabilities, and officials in some of these agencies said they can serve a much smaller population. For example, 57 percent (12 of 21) of agencies for the blind reported providing job exploration counseling to more students, compared to 83 percent (25 of 30) of combined agencies and 91 percent (20 of 22) of general agencies since WIOA enactment. Similarly, 67 percent (14 of 21) of agencies for the blind reported providing work-based learning experiences to more students, compared to 83 percent (25 of 30) for combined agencies and 86 percent (19 of 22) for general agencies.[20] Officials in some of these agencies for the blind and from the National Council of State Agencies for the Blind (NCSAB) told us in interviews that agencies for the blind have far fewer potentially eligible students they could serve compared to other types of agencies. For example, officials we interviewed with Idaho's Commission for the Blind and Visually Impaired said that Idaho has only 40 students being provided pre-employment transition services. In contrast, the Idaho Division of Vocational Rehabilitation reportedly provided at least one pre-employment transition service to approximately 700 students in a one-year period.

The ability of agencies for the blind to serve more students may also be restricted because they are not able to provide pre-employment transition services to younger students in some cases, according to officials with NCSAB and Idaho's Commission for the Blind and Visually Impaired. NCSAB officials told us that state VR agencies have traditionally provided VR services to youth who are blind or visually impaired at younger ages compared to general agencies that serve youth with other types of disabilities. The ages at which students may be provided pre-employment transition services varied by agency, based on responses to our survey, but the most common

---

[19] GAO, *Supplemental Security Income: SSA Could Strengthen Its Efforts to Encourage Employment for Transition-Age Youth,* GAO-17-485 (Washington, D.C.: May 17, 2017).

[20] One general agency did not answer this survey question.

age range reported across all types of agencies was 14 to 21 years old. According to Education officials, as a result of WIOA, two agencies in the same state must agree on a common age range during which students can be provided pre-employment transition services. Most agencies in states with two VR agencies responding to our survey (35 of 44) reported agreeing on an age range for receiving preemployment transition services.[21] NCSAB officials said that in some cases agencies for the blind have had to raise the minimum age at which they would begin providing services to students. Officials with Idaho's Commission for the Blind and Visually Impaired, for example, said they would prefer to begin services at younger ages because their agency has the resources to do so. However, officials with Idaho's Division of Vocational Rehabilitation said they do not have the resources to provide pre-employment transition services to the relatively large number of students with disabilities at a younger age.

Most State Vocational Rehabilitation Agencies Reported Building Administrative Capacity

State VR agencies reported taking a range of actions to build their administrative capacity to implement pre-employment transition services. These actions included building staff capacity and expanding contracts with services providers.

- Building staff capacity. Most state VR agencies reported building staff capacity to facilitate and carry out the requirements of pre-employment transition services by:
  - Establishing a new specialist position. More than half (45 of 74) of VR agencies reported in our survey establishing at least one new transition specialist position specifically for pre-employment

[21] Of the respondents from agencies in states with two agencies, 6 of 44 reported that the agreement was in-progress. Three of 44 reported that they had not agreed. In four of the states we surveyed (8 agencies), the 2 agencies in the same state reported differently on whether they had agreed, an agreement was in-progress, or they had not agreed on an age range with the other VR agency.

transition services. For example, the Idaho Division of Vocational Rehabilitation reported establishing this position and officials told us that they hired a specialist who was previously the transition coordinator for the state's educational agency. In written comments on our survey, a respondent from another state commented that their agency has hired 20 pre-employment transition services specialists to provide the five required activities. Officials we interviewed from Maryland's Division of Rehabilitation Services said they added six salaried positions dedicated to providing pre-employment transition services. Another agency responding to our survey reported dedicating a supervisor and 15 percent of their counselors exclusively to this purpose.

- Training staff. All 74 state VR agencies reported providing training on pre-employment transition services to their staff. For example, in written comments, one agency reported developing training tools for its counselors, such as answers to frequently asked questions, posting guidance on its intranet, and having WINTAC provide training.

- Expanding contracts and agreements with service providers. In addition to being provided by state VR agency staff, pre-employment services can be offered through a variety of methods and service providers, and many state VR agencies reported entering into new or additional contracts with service providers or expanding contracts with existing providers. Pre-employment transition services can be provided directly by state VR agency staff or through agreements with third parties, such as community rehabilitation programs, independent living agencies, public colleges and universities, and school districts.[22] In our survey, 62 of 74 agencies reported entering into new or additional contracts with third-party providers to provide pre-employment transition services. Officials we interviewed from three of four state VR agencies said they either established or expanded

[22] See 29 U.S.C. § 733(a).

existing contracts and agreements. For example, officials from the Illinois Department of Human Service, Division of Rehabilitation Services told us that after the enactment of WIOA, they expanded arrangements with independent living centers and initiated a new program that provides students with work experiences. Agencies reported several examples of approaches using third parties:

- establishing contracts with community rehabilitation programs to provide work experiences,
- partnering with independent living agencies to work with youth on self-advocacy,
- entering into provider agreements with local workforce centers to assist with providing job preparation and a paid work experience,
- developing programs with public colleges and universities focused on financial literacy and self-advocacy, and
- contracting with individual school districts to deliver services in the school environment.

States Reported Challenges Using Reserved Funds, Updating Interagency Agreements, Among Others, and Reported Needing More Assistance from Education

Fewer Than Half of States Reported Using All Reserved Funds, and Some Reported a Need for More Information on Allowable Costs

Twenty-one of 56 states (50 states, 5 territories, and the District of Columbia) reported using the full amount of grant funds they reserved for pre-employment transition services for students with disabilities for fiscal year 2016, according to the most recent full year of data available from Education (see Figure 4).

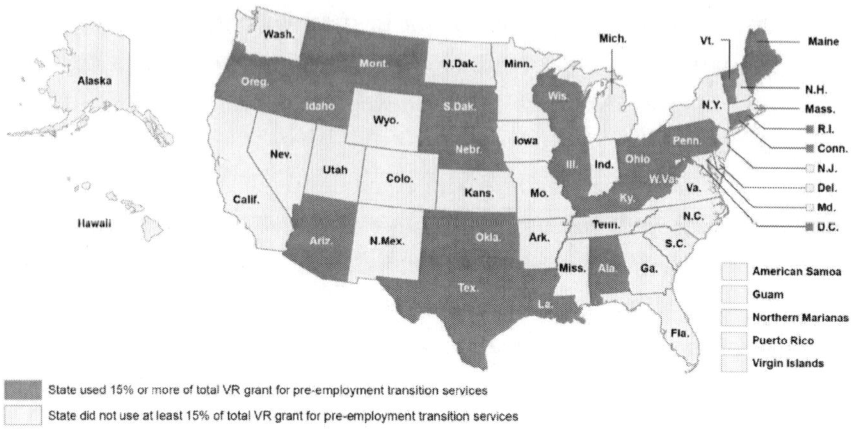

Source: GAO presentation of data reported by states to the U.S. Department of Education. | GAO-18-502.

Figure 4. Reported Use of Funds Reserved for Pre-Employment Transition Services for Students with Disabilities, by State, Fiscal Year 2016.

In aggregate, states reportedly expended approximately $357 million out of the approximately $465 million reserved (about $108 million less than the target) for fiscal year 2016. For fiscal year 2015, states reportedly expended approximately $324 million on pre-employment transition services out of the approximately $453 million reserved for that purpose (about $130 million less than the target).

Results from our 2017 survey of state VR agencies revealed similar trends: Fewer than half the 74 agencies reported that they used at least 15 percent of their VR grant allotment each year. Thirty-two of the 74 agencies responding to our survey reported using the minimum required 15 percent of federal VR grant funds reserved for the provision of preemployment transition services for fiscal years 2016 and 2017.[23] For fiscal year 2015, 25 agencies reported using the required 15 percent minimum reserved funds.[24]

Officials we interviewed in two of four state VR agencies and officials in all three discussion groups explained that some of the services they generally provided to participants in the VR program are not allowable for the funds reserved for pre-employment transition services. These expenditures included transportation, tuition, and others associated with individualized services. For example, officials in Maryland's Division of Rehabilitation Services told us that transportation costs for students to get to the place where the services are provided are not covered. VR agency officials in two of our discussion groups told us that assistive technology, such as hearing aids, could not be paid for with the 15 percent of funds reserved for pre-employment transition services. In another group, participants said that some expenditures, such as tuition or for the services of a job coach to help students with the most significant disabilities, could not be paid with reserved funds. In information provided with the regulations, Education stated that it does not have the statutory authority to allow these expenditures to be paid for with the funds reserved for pre-employment transition services and these services must be paid with other VR funds.

When it promulgated its final regulations, Education noted that state VR agencies would experience challenges in using their funds because many of the services provided to students with disabilities prior to WIOA's enactment would not qualify as pre-employment transition services. Education reviewed past expenditures for a subset of students and estimated that 82 percent of state VR agencies' reported purchases for those students would not meet the statutory definition of pre-employment services under WIOA. Education concluded that states would have to reach a larger number of students with disabilities in order to meet the spending

---

[23] We did not assess states' compliance with WIOA or Education's funding requirements with our analysis. States may expend some of these funds in the next fiscal year, as they are allowed to carry over funds awarded in a fiscal year for which they have provided a nonfederal match to the subsequent fiscal year to be obligated and expended in that subsequent year. Moreover, Education noted that states with two VR agencies may still meet the requirement to reserve and expend funds if their combined expenses meet or exceed the 15 percent requirement.

[24] Those who reported spending the 15 percent minimum requirement of their VR grant included all types of agencies (combined, general, and blind).

requirement and that state VR agencies would need to develop and implement aggressive strategies to expend these funds in these initial years of implementation.

According to WINTAC officials, state VR agency officials are commonly unclear about what kinds of activities they can provide using the funds reserved for pre-employment transition services. For instance, they said that states must make required activities (e.g., work-based learning experiences and self-advocacy) available to all students with disabilities before providing authorized activities (e.g., model projects, partnerships), in accordance with WIOA. However, state officials have commonly interpreted that to mean that all students must actually receive the required activities before the agency can begin providing other activities, according to WINTAC officials. WINTAC officials explained that states may have been conducting authorized or coordination activities without knowing these activities could be paid for with the reserved funds.

None of the state VR agency officials we interviewed said they had yet moved beyond providing required activities to providing authorized activities. Officials from two of the agencies we interviewed told us they were in the process of planning authorized activities. For example, officials with the Idaho Division of Vocational Rehabilitation said they were completing an assessment of their needs, which would help them plan authorized activities. Officials we interviewed from the other two agencies—the Idaho Commission for the Blind and Visually Impaired and the Illinois Division of Rehabilitation Services—said they did not have the resources to provide authorized activities or were unsure about how to properly transition from required to authorized activities under the current guidance.

Education communicated with states on broad requirements but provided little detailed information directly to states on the allowable use of funds reserved for pre-employment transition services. Education provided information when it promulgated final regulations, in grant award notifications, on its website, and in presentations at conferences. In each of these formats, Education described activities on which states could not spend funds, but provided little detailed information on what expenditures are allowed.

- Regulations: Education's final regulations restate many provisions in WIOA, including the prohibition on using any of the reserved funds for administrative costs. In responding to comments it received on its proposed regulations, Education provided examples of services that commenters requested would be considered pre-employment transition services, such as, postsecondary education, on-the-job supports, job coaching, travel expenses, and uniforms. In information provided with the regulations, Education explained that it had no statutory authority to expand or limit the pre-employment transition services listed in WIOA. Education stated that a state VR agency can allocate costs associated with staff time spent providing preemployment transition services, including an employee's salary and fringe benefits, to the funds reserved for pre-employment transition services.[25] However, Education did not provide additional information on what specific types of expenditures states were permitted to spend funds on in providing pre-employment transition services as required by WIOA.
- Grant award notification: The notification that accompanies each state's VR grant award lists the three sets of activities for which the reserved money can be used: required, authorized, and coordination; it lists each of the activities as they are listed in WIOA. It also discusses the prohibition on using any of the reserved funds for administrative costs. It does not list or describe what specific expenditures the reserved funds can be used for to undertake each of the listed activities.
- Education's website: A list of frequently asked questions on Education's website outlines the requirements of WIOA and

[25] In promulgating final regulations, Education noted that it has been its long-standing policy that staff-related costs, including salaries, fringe benefits, and travel, incurred while providing vocational rehabilitation services constitute service costs, not administrative costs. See 81 Fed. Reg. 55,630, 55,702 (Aug. 19, 2016).

explains that the reserved funds must only be used to provide pre-employment transition services as listed in WIOA. Similar to the regulations, the website explains that the total costs of an employee's salary and fringe benefits may be allocated to the reserved funds if that employee is providing only pre-employment transition services to students with disabilities but does not include additional detail for any other expenditures.

- Presentation materials: In one set of presentation materials, Education provided an example of a potential allowable expenditure for one of the required activities, work-based learning. It did not include information on allowable expenditures for the other four required activities, or any of the nine authorized activities. In another set of presentation materials, Education provided examples of services for each of the five required pre-employment transition services activities. According to Education officials, these examples would be allowable expenditures.

Education, however, provided the most detailed information through WINTAC. WINTAC's website provided answers to some specific questions on the use of funds reserved for pre-employment transition services. In one set of frequently asked questions, WINTAC included a list of 28 questions with detailed answers, including what specific expenditures may be charged to the reserved funds. For example, based upon guidance issued by RSA, the website explains that reserved funds may be used to pay for auxiliary aids and services, such as interpreters, if they are directly related to one of the five required pre-employment transition services activities. However, the reserved funds may not be used to pay for the costs of foreign language interpreters because they are not an auxiliary aid or serve that is required due to the individual's disability. WINTAC's website also included answers provided by Education on 13 other frequently asked questions. Information included that reserved funds cannot be used to pay for the cost of an assessment to determine whether a student met the definition of a student with a disability; they can be used to pay for items required by an employer for work-based learning activities.

Some state VR agencies we surveyed and those that participated in one of our three discussion groups said they would like more detailed information directly from Education. Seven survey respondents reported that they would like Education to provide answers to their specific questions. In one discussion group, participants noted that when states approach WINTAC with a new question, the technical assistance center sometimes needs to obtain the answer from Education. This process can be inefficient at times. In addition, the answer may not be broadly shared with all the states, limiting its benefit, whereas information issued directly from Education could help communicate the answer more efficiently and broadly. One survey respondent reported, for example, that guidance varied by source—training, Education's RSA staff, or technical assistance center websites—and said that Education should provide all state VR agencies with the same information at the same time.

According to standards for federal internal control, management should communicate externally through reporting lines so that external parties can help the entity achieve its objectives and address related risks.[26] Management should also periodically evaluate its methods of communication so it has the appropriate tools to communicate quality information throughout and outside of the entity on a timely basis.[27] Education officials said that during fiscal years 2015 and 2016, states were unclear about allowable expenditures using reserved funds, and that they plan to clarify guidance as they learn about the issues from states during their monitoring. According to Education officials, they respond to issues that need clarification and provide answers to questions as part of formal monitoring visits or through other communications with state agencies. Education officials said they expect to complete a round of monitoring visits to all states by the end of fiscal year 2021. However, an Education official said they have no timeframe for providing further information on allowable costs to states. With better information on timeframes for when

---

[26] GAO, *Standards for Internal Control in the Federal Government,* GAO-14-704G (Washington, D.C.: September 2014), 62.

[27] GAO-14-704G, 63.

this information will be provided, states would be able to better plan their use of the remaining funds reserved for preemployment transition services.

State VR and Educational Agencies Have Begun Collaborating through Joint Training and Guidance, but Fewer Than Half Have Updated Their Interagency Agreements

Most state VR agencies (61 of 74) that responded to our survey reported providing training on pre-employment transition services along with their state's educational agency since WIOA's enactment in 2014. Joint training may help coordination between state VR and educational agencies, as state VR officials participating in our discussion groups said that some educators were not familiar with pre-employment transition services. Similarly, an official we interviewed from Idaho's state educational agency said it was common in the past for teachers and VR counselors not to know one another. Joint trainings provided to VR staff and teachers have improved these relationships, and teachers can invite VR counselors to students' IEP meetings, the official said.

Joint training includes staff presentations at conferences and participation in other training sessions. For example, officials we interviewed from the Idaho Division of Vocational Rehabilitation said their transition coordinator has given presentations to education directors around the state about changes resulting from WIOA and how the inclusion of pre-employment transition services can affect special education for the school districts. In written comments on our survey, one agency reported that it co-sponsors an annual conference with VR, special education, developmental services, and other public and private entities. During this conference, they plan how to improve services for students with disabilities.

About one-third of state VR agencies (23 of 74) reported issuing joint guidance with their state's educational agency, a recommended practice according to WINTAC. The other two-thirds of survey respondents reported that joint guidance was either in progress (27 of 74) or that they had not issued such guidance (23 of 74).[28] Joint guidance can include written policies and procedures that are created by and provided to state VR and educational agency staff. For example, in written comments on our survey, one agency reported developing written policies and guidance for transition counselors that the state educational agency endorses and provides to special education staff. In Maryland, VR and special education officials told us that they issued guidance through jointly created materials on pre-employment transition services.

Less than half the state VR agencies that responded to our survey (34 of 74) reported updating their interagency agreement with their state's educational agency, which is intended to facilitate collaboration and coordination on delivery of pre-employment transition services. The majority of agencies reported that their agreement is either in progress (37 of 74) or not yet updated (3 of 74). These required agreements outline how VR agencies and schools will plan and coordinate service provision, provide for each agency's responsibilities, including financial responsibilities, and provide for student outreach procedures, among other things.[29]

Discussion group participants and CSAVR representatives emphasized the value of completing their interagency agreements with the state educational agency. In one group, officials whose agencies had completed their agreements said they are essential for state VR agencies to provide services in schools. Participants in another discussion group explained that once they have a state-level agreement in place, they can discuss what services school districts need for students and then determine how to provide those services. According to state educational agency officials we interviewed, Individuals with Disabilities Education Act (IDEA) requirements are similar to requirements for pre-employment transition services, and they need to coordinate with VR officials at both the state and local levels to agree on each agency's assigned tasks and expectations. These officials said state VR and educational agencies should coordinate funding to make services available where they are needed and to complement each other's transition efforts. Illinois's

[28] One survey respondent did not answer the question.
[29] See 29 U.S.C. § 721(a)(11)(D).

agreement, for example, specifies that the state educational agency is responsible for providing outreach, guidance, and coordination to local educational agencies regarding the provision of pre-employment transition services. According to the agreement, Illinois's VR agency is responsible for providing pre-employment transition services, both directly and through cooperative agreements with local educational agencies, and for providing written information to the state educational agency regarding services available to students with disabilities. Officials we interviewed with CSAVR said state VR agencies that have made progress in developing their interagency agreements with state educational agencies tend to be more successful in implementing pre-employment transition services. According to Education officials, Education provides guidance and technical assistance on interagency agreements to states as part of Education's monitoring or when asked by states. Education officials said they provide technical assistance during periodic monitoring visits, which are currently limited to about 10 states per year from fiscal years 2017-2021; by helping state VR agencies develop policies and procedures; and by making sure pre-employment transition services are coordinated with the state educational agency and through interagency agreements. According to Education officials, there is no statutory provision authorizing Education to identify states that have not updated their interagency agreement. Education officials said they do not collect information from state VR agencies on the status of these agreements except when they conduct monitoring visits in specific states. In addition, Education officials said that when monitoring, they may meet with state educational agency partners to help them understand the new components of preemployment transition services in an agreement, or they may refer the state agencies to WINTAC or NTACT resources. Providing assistance during monitoring may be helpful for some states. However, given that less than half of state VR agencies we surveyed reported updating and finalizing their agreements and Education officials say they will take another three years to complete this round of monitoring, additional action by Education may be needed to raise awareness among the remaining states about the importance of these agreements to help states coordinate services to students with disabilities. Additional action could include, for example, conducting earlier state outreach or monitoring to assess state progress on finalizing the interagency agreements and offering technical assistance when appropriate.

However, Education officials said there is no requirement that state educational agencies provide pre-employment transition services to meet their obligations to IDEA-eligible students with disabilities under part B of the Individuals with Disabilities Education Act.[30] As a result, WINTAC and participants in our discussion groups explained that it can be difficult to get state educational agencies to work with state VR agencies to update interagency agreements.

Education officials said that WIOA requires state VR agencies to update these interagency agreements to include preemployment transition services but they do not track their completion because states are not required to report when the agreements are finalized. Moreover, Education officials said they have heard from states that some reasons that interagency agreements are not specifically updated are that the agreements are written broadly enough so that they can remain in effect when there are additional changes to the law, the details of actual practices are rarely reflected in the high level of an interagency agreement, and that modifications to agreements are time-consuming and would not result in changes to the interagency coordination practice.

Without an updated agreement between the state VR and educational agencies, efforts to collaborate on pre-employment transition services may be hindered. Officials with the National Technical Assistance Center on Transition (NTACT) told us that some of the state agencies for which they provided in-depth technical assistance were not working closely together. Officials from two of the three state educational agencies we interviewed said they viewed pre-employment transition services as

---

[30] The Individuals with Disabilities Education Act (IDEA) does not include language pertaining to pre-employment transition services.

primarily the responsibility of the VR agency. State VR officials in all three of our discussion groups said they have experienced coordination challenges, including difficulty determining each agency's responsibilities for providing pre-employment transition services, obtaining data needed to identify and provide services to students, and determining which agency will pay for which services, among other challenges. Interagency agreements can help to address these types of issues.

Federal internal controls recommend that management communicate with and obtain information to identify, analyze, and respond to risks related to achieving defined objectives, such as those that can arise from new laws and regulations.[31] Moreover, we found in prior work that it is important to establish ways to operate across agency boundaries, with measures such as developing common terminology and fostering open lines of communication.[32] A lack of collaboration between state VR and educational agencies increases the risk that some students will not successfully transition from school to post-school activities. In addition, our prior work has identified lack of collaboration among and between federal agencies and state and local governments as a challenge to effective grant implementation.[33]

Interagency agreements are intended to serve as a mechanism related to collaboration practices, which include defining a common outcome, establishing joint strategies, and agreeing on roles and responsibilities of each agency. By taking additional steps, such as discussing the benefits of finalizing interagency agreements, and reminding states of existing technical assistance resources pertaining to updating and finalizing interagency agreements, Education would help raise awareness about the importance of the agreements and be better positioned to help states efficiently and effectively coordinate services to students with disabilities.

---

[31] GAO-14-704G, 62.

[32] GAO, *Managing for Results: Key Considerations for Implementing Interagency Collaborative Mechanisms,* GAO-12-1022 (Washington, D.C.: September 27, 2012).

[33] GAO, *Grants to State and Local Governments: An Overview of Federal Funding Levels and Selected Challenges,* GAO-12-1016 (Washington, D.C: September 25, 2012).

States Reported That Best Practices Would Be Useful to Them in Implementing Services and Could Help Them Address Challenges

Most state VR agencies (63 of 74) that responded to our survey reported that additional assistance with identifying best practices would be useful to their agencies.[34] Similarly, state VR officials in all three of our discussion groups spoke to the need for Education to develop and disseminate best practices to help states, for example, comply with program requirements. WIOA requires Education to highlight best state practices on pre-employment transition services.[35] Best practices may also help states address the challenges they reported facing in implementing and administering pre-employment transition services for students with disabilities, such as (1) coordinating with state educational agencies, (2) using VR resources more efficiently and effectively to help states balance providing pre-employment services with the full VR program, and (3) collecting data on services provided, and (4) updating data tracking systems.

- Coordinating service delivery with state educational agencies. Over half (41 of 74) of state VR agencies reported in our survey that additional assistance on coordinating with state educational agencies would be useful for them.[36] Similarly, officials from all three state educational agencies we interviewed said they would like additional assistance on interagency collaboration. Officials with NTACT told us that some of the state agencies for which they provided in-depth technical assistance were not working closely together. Officials from two of the three state educational agencies we interviewed said they viewed pre-employment transition

---

[34] Seven survey respondents answered "no," three answered "don't know," and one did not answer this question.

[35] See 29 U.S.C. § 733(e) ("The Secretary shall support designated State agencies providing services under this section, highlight best State practices, and consult with other Federal agencies to advance the goals of this section").

[36] The remaining state VR agencies reported in our survey that additional assistance on coordinating with state educational agencies would not be useful (28 of 74), "don't know" (4 of 74), or did not answer this question (1 of 74).

services as primarily the responsibility of the VR agency. State VR officials in all three of our discussion groups said they have experienced coordination challenges, including difficulty determining each agency's responsibilities for providing pre-employment transition services, obtaining data needed to identify and provide services to students, and determining which agency will pay for which services, among other challenges. An official we interviewed from the Idaho Department of Education said it would be helpful to have more clearly defined roles, obligations, and means of sharing data between the state-level agencies. In written responses to our survey, one respondent said having examples of highly successful collaborations between a state educational agency and state VR agencies would be helpful. According to Education's guidance, a student's transition from school to post-school activities is a shared responsibility and coordination and collaboration between the state VR and educational agencies is essential. However, according to information Education provided with the regulations, while some have sought clarification and additional guidance in this area, Education determined that decisions on agencies' responsibilities must be made at the state level to allow states maximum flexibility allowed under the law. In the absence of more specific guidelines for how state agencies should collaborate, best practices from other states could provide helpful examples.

- Balancing pre-employment transition services with VR services. Several state VR agencies in both our written survey responses and in discussion groups noted that by increasing services mandated for pre-employment transition services for students, they have had to reduce VR services to adults, which has made it difficult to balance the two programs. In issuing its final regulations, Education acknowledged that reserving funds would decrease amounts available for the full VR program, resulting in a transfer of benefits from individuals historically served by VR to students with disabilities in need of transition services. According to state VR directors with the National Council of State Agencies for the

Blind (NCSAB), agencies for the blind have had to restrict VR services while also not being able to use all of the funds reserved for pre-employment transition services for students with disabilities because VR services cannot be paid with reserved funds. Most state VR agencies that completed our survey (50 of 74) reported that balancing pre-employment transition services with other vocational rehabilitation services was moderately difficult, very difficult, or extremely difficult during federal fiscal year 2017.[37]

- Collecting data. Data collection was one of the top challenges identified by state VR agencies in our survey, with 48 of 74 reporting that collecting data on the provision of pre-employment transition services was moderately difficult, very difficult, or extremely difficult during fiscal year 2017. Prior to WIOA, agencies collected and reported data only on individuals who had applied and enrolled in the VR program. For pre-employment transition services, agencies now collect data on who provided and received each of the five required activities, including for individuals who have not submitted a VR application. State VR officials in two of our three discussion groups said that they have experienced challenges collecting sensitive information (such as social security numbers) for minors and collecting data on individuals for group services. Officials in one of the three discussion groups also said that these problems are particularly significant when trying to collect information on potentially eligible students for whom they do not have open VR cases. These students could include all those with an IEP and those that receive accommodations in school based on their disability, among others.
- Updating data tracking systems. Updating data systems was also one of the top challenges reported in our survey, and was cited as an additional administrative burden by state VR officials in our discussion groups. Specifically, 53 of 74 state VR agencies reported

---

[37] The remaining state VR agencies reported in our survey that balancing pre-employment transition services with other vocational rehabilitation services was slightly difficult (20 of 74), not at all difficult (3 of 74), or "don't know" (1 of 74).

that it was moderately difficult, very difficult, or extremely difficult to update tracking systems to collect and report financial and service data on pre-employment transition services during fiscal year 2017. According to a state VR agency official we interviewed, updating that state's tracking system is difficult because data collected on pre-employment transition services—such as the type of service provider and how the service was provided—do not fit well into a case management system designed for the full VR program. Updating these tracking systems also created an additional administrative burden for VR agency staff, according to officials from all three discussion groups and three of the four state agencies that we interviewed. Officials in two of our three discussion groups said that they have one or more full-time staff members doing only administrative tasks or that they have had to hire additional staff to handle data tracking.

Education officials said that they plan to document and share best practices with states; however, they said the agency does not have a final written plan for managing these efforts because plans are still under discussion in light of inquiries received. Education officials said they are collecting information on state VR agencies' practices through monitoring and they are sharing this information with WINTAC—information that could be useful for sharing best practices across states—but a comprehensive summary of states' efforts will not be available until after Education officials conduct monitoring visits of all states by the end of fiscal year 2021. In addition, in a 2015 technical assistance circular, Education recommended that state VR agencies consult with other federal, state, and local agencies to identify best practices for providing pre-employment transition services to students and youth with a variety of disabilities. Education officials also said that they are looking for opportunities, such as webinars and conferences, to share information with states. However, Education does not have set timeframes and has not detailed the specific steps and activities for fully leveraging knowledge to address common challenges, or for finalizing and disseminating best practices. By doing so, Education would be better positioned to provide best practices information to state VR agencies to better serve students with disabilities who are transitioning from high school.

CONCLUSION

Pre-employment transition services are designed to help students with disabilities begin to identify career interests and move from high school to post-secondary education or employment. Using federal funding, state VR agencies reported that they have generally enhanced their services and staff capacity and begun to coordinate with state educational agencies. As a result, state VR agencies generally reported serving an increased number of students. However, most states reported they have not used all the funds reserved for pre-employment transition services or updated interagency agreements between state VR and educational agencies. Education has developed multiple forms of guidance and made presentations, either directly or through its technical assistance centers. Education officials said they plan to issue additional guidance as needed. However, without clear timeframes for the issuance of this guidance, states do not know when information will become available to help them make decisions on allowable expenditures for pre-employment transition services. As a result, opportunities may be missed to identify and serve all students who might be eligible, and unserved students could continue to face difficulties preparing for a future of meaningful post-secondary education or employment. In addition, agreements between state VR and educational agencies can help facilitate the effective coordination of and financial responsibility for services. Finally, WIOA requires Education to highlight best state practices for implementing pre-employment transition services. Developing a written plan with specific timeframes would help Education provide states with information on best practices, such as balancing service delivery between pre-employment transition services and other VR services and collecting data that other states may have successfully addressed.

Recommendations for Executive Action

We are making the following three recommendations to Education:

The Secretary of Education should establish timeframes for providing states with additional information on allowable expenditures of funds reserved for pre-employment transition services. (Recommendation 1)

The Secretary of Education should take additional steps to provide states assistance on updating and finalizing their interagency agreements with state educational agencies to include pre-employment transition services. These steps could include, for example, accelerating their efforts to discuss the benefits of finalizing interagency agreements, and reminding states of existing technical assistance resources pertaining to updating and finalizing interagency agreements. (Recommendation 2)

The Secretary of Education should develop a written plan with specific timeframes and activities for identifying and disseminating best practices that address, as appropriate, implementation challenges for preemployment transition services, such as those identified in this chapter. (Recommendation 3)

Agency Comments and Our Evaluation

We provided a draft of this chapter to Education for review and comment. Education's written comments are reproduced in appendix III. Education also provided technical comments, which we incorporated into our report where appropriate.

Education concurred with recommendation 1 and disagreed with recommendations 2 and 3 in the draft report.

With regard to recommendation 1, Education stated that it agreed and will establish projected timeframes for providing states with additional information on allowable expenditures for the provision of pre-employment transition services. Education also stated that it intends to provide states with additional information in at least two forums before the end of calendar year 2018 and to review and analyze previous guidance provided to states on allowable expenditures.

With regard to the draft report's recommendation 2, which called for Education to identify states that have not updated and finalized their interagency agreements to include pre-employment transition services, Education stated that it disagreed, in large part, because there is no statutory provision authorizing the agency to identify such states. However, Education is taking some steps as part of its ongoing monitoring of the VR program to provide assistance to states that have not updated their interagency agreements, which is consistent with the intention of our recommendation, but more could be done. Education stated that it will continue to offer and provide technical assistance if it becomes known through the onsite monitoring of the VR program or through other means that states have not updated their interagency agreements between VR agencies and state educational agencies. It also noted that the Rehabilitation Services Administration (RSA) and its Office of Special Education Programs will provide information related to sources of technical assistance, as appropriate, to VR agencies and state educational agencies. While these steps may be helpful, given the number of states that have not updated and finalized their agreements and the length of time Education officials say they will take to complete this round of monitoring where Education asks state VR agencies about these agreements, additional action by Education may be needed to help states more efficiently and effectively coordinate services to students with disabilities.

Education also wrote that while the Rehabilitation Act requires an interagency agreement, the Individuals with Disabilities Education Act does not contain a parallel requirement for state and local educational agencies with respect to the provision of pre-employment transition services or the incorporation of such discussion into the interagency agreement. In light of these differing requirements, as we state in our report, stakeholders with whom we spoke indicated it can be difficult to get state educational agencies to work with state VR agencies to update interagency agreements. Therefore, it is all the more important for Education to take additional action to engage with VR agencies regarding interagency agreements and to work closely with VR agencies as Education becomes aware of states that have not updated their agreements.

Education suggested a modified recommendation that removed reference to Education identifying states that have not updated and finalized their agreements. We modified the recommendation and the report to address Education's concerns about its authority to identify states. By taking additional steps, such as discussing the benefits of finalizing interagency agreements, and reminding states of existing technical assistance resources pertaining to updating and finalizing interagency agreements, Education would help raise awareness about the importance of the interagency agreements and be better positioned to help states efficiently and effectively coordinate services to students with disabilities.

With regard to recommendation 3, Education stated that it disagreed because it is premature to develop a timeline for the dissemination of best practices. Education stated that the identification of "best" practices, meaning those that are clearly supported by a body of evidence derived from valid and reliable research findings, is still emerging as states implement the requirements. Education suggested a modified recommendation that included planning for the dissemination of best practices identified by states as they become available. Education stated in its comments that as RSA identifies best practices through its monitoring and technical assistance activities, it will, in collaboration with its Office of Special Education Programs, consider when and how best to disseminate this information to state VR and educational agencies. With regard to including specific timeframes and activities in a written plan, by detailing the specific steps Education is taking and plans to take along with the amount of time it expects them to take, Education would be better positioned to complete those steps in a timely manner and meet the statutory requirement that Education highlight best state practices and support state agencies.

Sincerely yours,
Elizabeth H. Curda
Director, Education, Workforce and Income Security

APPENDIX I: OBJECTIVES, SCOPE, AND METHODOLOGY

The objectives of this chapter are to examine (1) the steps states have reported taking to implement pre-employment transition services, and (2) the implementation challenges, if any, states reported facing, and how the Department of Education (Education) has addressed them.

To address these objectives, we reviewed federal laws and regulations, and Education's guidance and technical assistance documents, including circulars, policy directives, and transition guides. We also reviewed expenditure data reported by state vocational rehabilitation (VR) agencies to Education for fiscal years 2015 and 2016, the most recent full years of data available. To assess the reliability of the data, we interviewed Education officials about their collection of the data and their opinion of the data's quality, completeness, and accuracy. We also electronically tested the data for any obvious errors. We determined that the data were reliable for the purposes of our review. We interviewed representatives from the Council of State Administrators of Vocational Rehabilitation (CSAVR) and the National Council of State Agencies for the Blind. In addition, we interviewed officials from Education's Office of Special Education and Rehabilitation Services, Rehabilitation Services Administration, Office of Special Education Programs, and the Workforce Innovation Technical Assistance Center and National Technical Assistance Center on Transition—two technical assistance centers funded by Education.

Survey of State Vocational Rehabilitation (VR) Agencies

To address both of the objectives, we conducted a survey of all 79 state VR agencies from October through December 2017. Seventy-four of the 79 agencies (94 percent) responded. The survey questionnaire included open-ended and closed-ended questions about agencies' efforts to train staff, update interagency agreements, expand services to students with disabilities, and other issues. We took steps to minimize the potential errors that may be introduced by the practical difficulties of conducting any survey. Because we selected the entire population of VR agencies for our survey, our estimates are not subject to sampling error. We conducted pretests of the draft questionnaire with three agencies in the population and made revisions to reduce the possibility of measurement error from differences in how questions were interpreted and the sources of information available to respondents.

We reviewed state officials' submitted survey responses and conducted follow-up, as necessary, to determine that their responses were complete, reasonable, and sufficiently reliable for the purposes of this chapter. A second independent analyst checked the accuracy of all computer analyses we performed to minimize the likelihood of errors in data processing. We made multiple follow-up attempts during the survey with agencies that had not yet responded. The five agencies that did not respond had smaller values, on average, on three characteristics related to size, than those that did respond.[38] The nonrespondents tended to be smaller than respondent agencies. The sums totals for each of these three characteristics across the five nonresponding agencies comprised less than 1 percent of the totals for the population, suggesting a lower possibility of material error in our results from nonresponse.[39]

Interviews and Discussion Groups with State VR Agencies

For more in-depth information on both of the objectives, we conducted interviews and held discussion groups. We conducted interviews with

[38] These three characteristics were: eligible service populations, numbers served, and grant totals. The nonresponding agencies did not materially differ from responding agencies across the fourth known characteristic—the percentage of their state populations in urban areas. These characteristics may or may not be related to the nature of agency answers to some survey questions.

[39] Nonresponse error can result when a survey fails to capture information from all cases sampled, or in this case, the population. Nonresponse reduces the precision of estimates due to the smaller number of observations, and may introduce bias if those not responding, in the aggregate, would have given materially different answers to a question compared to those who did respond.

officials in Idaho, Illinois, and Maryland. For each state, we interviewed state VR officials and state educational agency officials. We selected these states for variety using the following criteria: size of the special education population (large, medium, and small); state agency organization, for example, whether the VR agency was organized under the state's educational or other department; and whether the state had a second agency for serving individuals who are blind or visually impaired.[40]

We convened three discussion groups with state VR agency directors or their designated officials, with a total of 39 participants from 29 separate agencies (10 to 12 agencies represented per discussion group). These discussion groups took place during a conference of state VR directors in November 2017 in Greenville, South Carolina. To select participants, we worked with the conference organizer, CSAVR, to send invitations for our discussion groups to all conference attendees. We additionally included a question in our survey asking respondents whether they would like to participate in discussion groups at the conference, and contacted those who responded affirmatively via phone and email. We moderated each discussion to keep participants focused on the specified issues within discussion timeframes.

Criteria Applied

To assess Education's efforts to address state VR agencies' challenges in providing pre-employment transition services, we applied standards for internal control in the federal government.[41] Specifically, we applied principle 15 related to communicating with external parties.[42] In addition, regarding Education's assistance to state VR agencies' efforts to update interagency agreements with state educational agencies, we also applied key

---

[40] Using data from Education on the number of individuals ages 12-21 receiving special education and related services in each state, we determined 30,000 and fewer individuals to be "small"; between 30,000 and 100,000 to be "medium"; and 100,000 or more to be "large."

[41] GAO, *Standards for Internal Control in the Federal Government,* GAO-14-704G (Washington, D.C.: September 2014).

[42] GAO-14-704G, 62-63.

considerations for implementing interagency collaborative mechanisms that we have previously identified.[43]

We conducted this performance audit from February 2017 to September 2018 in accordance with generally accepted government auditing standards. Those standards require that we plan and perform the audit to obtain sufficient, appropriate evidence to provide a reasonable basis for our findings and conclusions based on our audit objectives. We believe that the evidence obtained provides a reasonable basis for our findings and conclusions based on our audit objectives.

APPENDIX II: WIOA AUTHORIZED ACTIVITIES FOR PRE-EMPLOYMENT TRANSITION SERVICES

Table 2. The Nine Authorized Pre-employment Transition Services Activities under the Workforce Innovation and Opportunity Act (WIOA)

Activity	Description
Independence and inclusion	Implementing effective strategies to increase the likelihood of independent living and inclusion in communities and competitive integrated workplaces.
Strategy development	Developing and improving strategies for individuals with intellectual disabilities and individuals with significant disabilities to live independently, participate in postsecondary education experiences, and obtain and retain competitive integrated employment.
Service provider instruction	Providing instruction to vocational rehabilitation counselors, school transition personnel, and other persons supporting students with disabilities.
Information dissemination	Disseminating information about innovative, effective, and efficient approaches to achieve the goals of pre-employment transition services.
Local coordination	Coordinating activities with transition services provided by local educational agencies under the Individuals with Disabilities Education Act.

[43] GAO, *Managing for Results: Key Considerations for Implementing Interagency Collaborative Mechanisms,* GAO-12-1022 (Washington, D.C.: September 27, 2012).

Activity	Description
Evidence-based improvements	Applying evidence-based findings to improve policy, procedure, practice, and the preparation of personnel, in order to better achieve the goals of pre-employment transition services.
Model projects	Developing model transition demonstration projects.
Partnerships	Establishing or supporting multistate or regional partnerships involving states, local education agencies, designated state units, developmental disability agencies, private businesses, or other participants to achieve the goals of pre-employment transition services.
Traditionally unserved populations	Disseminating information and strategies to improve the transition to postsecondary activities by individuals who are members of traditionally unserved populations.

Source: WIOA | GAO-18-502.

Appendix III: Comments from the United States Department of Education

UNITED STATES DEPARTMENT OF EDUCATION
OFFICE OF SPECIAL EDUCATION AND REHABILITATIVE SERVICES

THE ASSISTANT SECRETARY

August 9, 2018

Elizabeth H. Curda
Director
Education, Workforce and
Income Security Issues
U.S. Government Accountability Office
441 G Street, NW
Washington, DC 20548

Dear Ms. Curda:

I am writing in response to the recommendations made in the U.S. Government Accountability Office (GAO) draft report, "Students With Disabilities: Additional Information From Education Could Help States Provide Pre-Employment Transition Services" (GAO-18-502). We appreciate the opportunity to comment on the draft report on behalf of the U.S. Department of Education (Department).

Over the past several decades the provision of transition services has been, and continues to be, a shared responsibility between State educational agencies (SEA) and State vocational rehabilitation (VR) agencies in each State.

Section 614(d)(1)(A)(i)(VIII) of the Individuals with Disabilities Education Act (IDEA) requires that the individualized education program (IEP) for each eligible student must address transition services requirements beginning not later than the first IEP to be in effect when the student turns 16, or younger if determined appropriate by the IEP Team, and must be updated annually thereafter. To meet IDEA's transition services requirements, the IEP must contain the instruction, services, and supports needed to assist the student to gain the skills and experiences necessary to reach his or her desired post-school goals to facilitate the student's movement from school to post-school activities. The Rehabilitation Act of 1973 (Rehabilitation Act) authorizes a continuum of services, such as pre-employment transition services, transition services, job placement services, other VR services, and supported employment services for eligible students and youth with disabilities, as appropriate, to secure meaningful careers. Each VR agency is required to describe in the VR services portion of its Unified or Combined State Plan its plans, policies, and procedures for the coordination between VR and education officials to facilitate the transition of students with disabilities from the receipt of educational services in school to the receipt of VR services, including pre-employment transition services. The IDEA does not include the concept of pre-employment transition services.

The draft report includes three recommendations to the Department. Our responses follow.

Recommendation 1: *The Secretary of Education should establish timeframes for providing states with additional information on allowable expenditures for use of funds reserved for pre-employment transition services.*

Response: The Department agrees with the Recommendation and will establish projected timeframes for providing States with additional information, as appropriate, that would describe the requirements, along with flexibilities available to the States when expending funds reserved for the provision of pre-employment transition services to students with disabilities under the VR program. As part of this effort, and already planned, given the needs expressed by States, the Department intends to provide States with additional information in at least two forums before the end of calendar year 2018. In addition, the Department intends to review and analyze previous guidance provided to States on allowable expenditures to determine what further clarification might be helpful to assist States in meeting statutory requirements related to the expenditure of funds reserved for the provision of pre-employment transition services.

Recommendation 2: *The Secretary of Education should identify states that have not updated and finalized their interagency agreements with state educational agencies to include pre-employment transition services and direct them to available technical assistance resources.*

Response: The Department disagrees, in large part, with the Recommendation given that there is no statutory provision authorizing the Department to identify those States that have not yet updated their interagency agreements with State educational agencies to incorporate a discussion of the provision of pre-employment transition services under the VR program. We recommend that the Recommendation be modified accordingly to read as follows:

The Secretary of Education should offer assistance to States that may benefit from assistance in updating and finalizing their interagency agreements with state educational agencies to include pre-employment transition services and advise them of available technical assistance resources.

The Department will continue to offer and provide technical assistance if it becomes known through the Rehabilitation Services Administration's (RSA) onsite monitoring of the VR program or through other means that States have not updated their interagency agreements between VR agencies and State educational agencies to discuss the provision of pre-employment transition services as required by section 101(a)(11)(D) of the Rehabilitation Act. RSA and the Office of Special Education Programs (OSEP) will also provide information related to sources of technical assistance, as appropriate, to VR agencies and SEAs. While the Rehabilitation Act requires an interagency agreement, it is important to note that the IDEA does not contain a parallel requirement for State and local educational agencies with respect to the provision of pre-employment transition services or the incorporation of such discussion into the interagency agreement. Section 612(a)(12) of the IDEA does require an interagency agreement or other mechanism for interagency coordination to ensure that services needed to ensure a free appropriate public education (FAPE), including transition services as defined in section 602(34) of the IDEA, are provided.

Recommendation 3: *The Secretary of Education should develop a written plan with specific time frames and activities for identifying and disseminating best practices that address, as appropriate, implementation challenges, such as those identified in this report.*

Response: The Department disagrees with this Recommendation as drafted because it is premature to develop a timeline for the dissemination of best practices. The implementation of the requirements for pre-employment transition services is an iterative process involving changes in two large service systems, VR and special education. Implementation challenges and some delays are to be expected. The provision of pre-employment transition services to students with disabilities involves a substantial reconfiguration of spending and delivery of services by VR agencies. Identification of "best" practices, meaning those that are clearly supported by a body of evidence derived from valid and reliable research findings, is still emerging as states implement the requirements. Thus, we recommend that the Recommendation be modified accordingly to read as follows:

The Secretary of Education should develop a written plan for disseminating best practices identified by States that address the delivery of pre-employment transition services as they become available, and include, as appropriate, State strategies for addressing implementation challenges, such as those identified in this report.

As RSA identifies best practices through its monitoring and technical assistance activities, it will, in collaboration with OSEP, consider when and how best to disseminate this information to State VR and educational agencies.

The Department appreciates the opportunity to review the draft report and comment on the recommendations. We also are enclosing technical comments for your consideration.

Sincerely,

Johnny W. Collett

Enclosure

APPENDIX IV: STAFF ACKNOWLEDGMENTS

In addition to Elizabeth H. Curda, Sara Schibanoff Kelly (Assistant Director), Paul Schearf (Analyst-In-Charge), Matthew Rabe, and Paul Wright made key contributions to this chapter. Also contributing to this chapter were James Bennett, Kristy Kennedy, Sheila R. McCoy, Thomas James, Jessica Orr, Sam Portnow, Carl Ramirez, Monica Savoy, Kate Van Gelder, Adam Wendel, and James Whitcomb.

In: Individuals with Disabilities
Editor: Aston Delgado
ISBN: 978-1-53615-030-8

Chapter 5

Special Minimum Wages for Workers with Disabilities: Frequently Asked Questions*

Benjamin Collins

Summary

The Fair Labor Standards Act (FLSA), as amended, sets the minimum wage for covered workers at $7.25 per hour. Section 14(c) of the FLSA permits certified employers to pay a worker with a disability that impairs the worker's productive capacity a special minimum wage (SMW). The SMW may be below the federal minimum wage but must be commensurate with the worker's productivity and the job's prevailing wage.

This short report answers common questions related to SMWs. It covers

- federal legislation that authorizes SMWs;
- how individuals qualify for SMWs;

---

* This is an edited, reformatted and augmented version of Congressional Research Service Publication No. R43468, dated December 16, 2016.

- how employers are certified to pay SMWs and how wage levels are set;
- data on employers that pay SMWs; and
- services that must be provided in conjunction with the payment of SMWs.

What Federal Law Regulates Minimum Wages?

The Fair Labor Standards Act (FLSA) establishes the minimum wage that must be paid to all covered workers.[1] Under current law, the federal minimum wage is $7.25 per hour.[2]

What Are the Provisions of the FLSA That Permit the Payment of Special Minimum Wages to Workers with Disabilities?

Section 14(c) of the FLSA permits the Secretary of Labor to issue certificates to employers that allow the certified employers to pay a worker "whose earning or productive capacity is impaired by age, physical or mental deficiency, or injury" wages that are less than the federal minimum wage.[3] The FLSA specifies that the intent of this policy is "to prevent curtailment of opportunities for employment" for workers with disabilities.

The FLSA and Department of Labor (DOL) guidance typically refer to a wage provided under Section 14(c) of the FLSA as a "special minimum wage" (SMW).

---

[1] The FLSA was enacted as P.L. 75-718. It is in the U.S. Code at 29 C.F.R. 201-219. For more information on the FLSA and minimum wage see CRS Report R42713, *The Fair Labor Standards Act (FLSA): An Overview* and CRS Report R43089, *The Federal Minimum Wage: In Brief.*

[2] Individual states may have a minimum wage that is higher than the federal minimum wage. In these states, employers must pay workers the higher state minimum wage. For more information on state minimum wages, see CRS Report R43792, *State Minimum Wages: An Overview*, by David H. Bradley.

[3] Policies may vary for workers employed under certain federal contracts.

WHAT CONDITIONS QUALIFY A WORKER FOR A SMW?

Workers with physical or mental disabilities, including disabilities related to age or injury, may be paid SMWs. However, the fact that a worker has a disability does not, by itself, qualify the worker to be paid a special minimum wage. The worker's "productive capacity" in the job must be measurably lower than the productive capacity of an experienced worker without a disability in a comparable job.

In the case of a worker age 24 or under, the worker must receive certain services prior to beginning work at an SMW. These services are designed to provide the worker with access to the competitive labor market before the worker accepts employment under a SMW certificate. These services and processes are described in more detail in the "What services must a youth with a disability receive prior to beginning work under an SMW certificate?" question later in this chapter.

HOW ARE WAGE LEVELS DETERMINED?

The wage of a worker employed under an SMW certificate must be commensurate with the worker's productivity and the prevailing wage for a worker without a disability in a comparable job in the same geographic area. The prevailing wage is not necessarily the minimum wage, but rather the "wage rate that is paid to an experienced worker not disabled for the work to be performed."[4]

For example, if the prevailing wage for a job is $10.00 per hour and the worker with a disability is determined to be 50% as productive as a worker without a disability in a comparable job, the hourly wage of the worker with a disability would be $5.00.[5] Notably, this process means that a worker with

[4] See 29 C.F.R. 525.10.

[5] For more information on prevailing wage rates and setting wages under Section 14(c), see 29 C.F.R. 525.9-10.

a disability whose production is the same as a worker without a disability must be paid the prevailing wage for the job.

Under current law, there is no wage floor for SMWs. Statute and regulations require employers that are certified to pay SMWs to review workers' productivity and the prevailing wage for the job at least every six months.[6]

How Does an Employer Become Certified to Pay SMWs?

Not all employers may pay SMWs. To be eligible to pay workers with disabilities SMWs, an employer must apply and be certified by DOL. The employer's application must describe the work that will be performed under the certificate and the prevailing wage surveys conducted by the employer.

Depending on the type of employer, certificates may be valid for one or two years. Renewal applications must provide information on workers currently paid SMW and information on productivity evaluations.[7]

How Many Employers Are Certified to Pay SMWs? What Are the Characteristics of Employers Who Are Certified to Pay SMWs?

As of July 1, 2016, there were 2,464 employers with issued SMW certificates.[8] *Table 1* presents data on the types of employers with SMW certificates issued. About 87% of issued certificates are held by Community

---

[6] Workers who are not paid an hourly wage must be reviewed and have their wages adjusted at least once every year. See 29 C.F.R. 529.9(b).

[7] For more information, see Wage and Hour Division Fact Sheet #39A, "How to Obtain a Certificate Authorizing the Payment of Special Minimum Wages to Workers with Disabilities under Section 14(c) of the Fair Labor Standards Act (FLSA)," http://www.dol.gov/whd/regs/compliance/whdfs39a.htm.

[8] An additional 124 employers were listed in the database as having pending certificates.

Rehabilitation programs. These programs may provide employment for groups of workers eligible for SMWs and are often referred to as "sheltered workshops."

Table 1. Employers with Issued Special Minimum Wage Certificates As of July 1, 2016

Type	Certificates
Community Rehabilitation Programs	2,142
School Work Experience Programs	153
Business Establishments	73
Hospitals or Institutions with Patient Workers	96
Total Certificates	2,464

Source: U.S. Department of Labor, Wage and Hour Division, Certificate Holders section of https://www.dol.gov/Whd/specialemployment/index.htm.

The glossary of the Wage and Hour Division *Field Operations Handbook* defines the type of certificate holders as follows:[9]

- *Community Rehabilitation Program*: Not-for-profit agencies that provide rehabilitation and employment opportunities for people with disabilities. Some may be affiliated with national organizations such as Goodwill Industries or The Arc, while others are private not-for-profit organizations located solely within their local communities.
- *School Work Experience Program*: A program in which a school system may place students with disabilities in jobs in the community at SMWs. Child labor restrictions still apply. The school applies for the certificate, which names the location at which the student(s) will be placed. Separate certificates are required for each business at which students are placed. The original certificate is maintained at the school and the school provides a copy to the business.

---

[9] See Section 64k00 of the Wage and Hour Division *Field Operations Handbook* at http://www.dol.gov/whd/FOH/ch64/64k00.htm.

- *Hospital or Institution*: A public or private, not-for-profit or for-profit, facility primarily engaged in providing residential care for the sick, the aged, or the mentally ill or retarded, including but not limited to nursing homes, intermediate care facilities, rest homes, convalescent homes, homes for the elderly and infirm, halfway houses, residential centers for drug addicts or alcoholics, and the like, whether licensed or not licensed. "Primarily" means that more than 50% of the facility's income is attributable to this residential care. These facilities may apply for Section 14(c) certificates to pay SMWs to "patient workers" (defined in next bullet).
- *Patient Worker*: A worker with a disability who is employed by a hospital or institution that provides residential care where such worker receives treatment or care. It does not matter whether such worker is a resident of the establishment or receiving care on an outpatient basis.

Business establishments are not defined in the handbook, but can generally be described as private, for-profit entities.

WHAT IS THE AVERAGE WAGE FOR WORKERS EMPLOYED UNDER A SMW CERTIFICATE?

Employers are not required to report the wage rates or productivity levels of workers employed under SMW certificates. As such, there is no regularly published source of wage levels.

HOW ARE THE SMW PROVISIONS OF THE FLSA ENFORCED?

The Wage and Hour Division (WHD) of DOL is responsible for administering and enforcing the FLSA, including the SMW provisions of

Section 14(c) of the FLSA. The WHD primarily enforces the law through investigations. If WHD investigators find a violation of the FLSA, the investigators recommend changes to bring the employer into compliance and oversee the payment of any back wage liability that may have been incurred.

WHD reviews of employers with SMW certificates include verifying that workers are eligible for SMWs (i.e., they have a disability that impairs their productive capabilities), reviewing that employers properly establish prevailing wages, and confirming that productivity reviews are conducted properly and in a timely manner as required by law. According to WHD, many of the most common violations relate to the proper establishment or updating of the prevailing wage.[10]

An individual employee may also petition to have his or her SMW reviewed. A petition is submitted to DOL and reviewed by an administrative law judge. DOL does not advocate on behalf of the employer or employee in these reviews.[11]

WHAT SERVICES MUST A YOUTH WITH A DISABILITY RECEIVE PRIOR TO BEGINNING WORK UNDER AN SMW CERTIFICATE?

The Workforce Innovation and Opportunity Act of 2014 (WIOA; P.L. 113-128) establishes a set of actions that a worker age 24 or under ("youth with a disability") must complete prior to beginning work under an SMW certificate.[12] Generally, the new requirements relate to a youth with a disability actively pursuing employment in the community earning a prevailing wage ("competitive integrated employment"). Once a worker has

---

[10] WHD lists the most common violations at http://www.dol.gov/elaws/esa/flsa/14c/20b.htm.

[11] Full review process is described in regulations at 29 C.F.R. 525.22.

[12] These provisions are in Section 511 of the Rehabilitation Act (29 U.S.C. 794g).

demonstrated and documented unsuccessful pursuit of competitive integrated employment, the worker may accept employment under an SMW certificate. The pre-employment requirements established by WIOA do not apply to workers over the age of 24 or workers who were employed under a SMW certificate prior to the law's effective date of July 22, 2016.[13]

Under the new provisions, a worker age 24 or under must complete *each* of the following actions prior to beginning work under an SMW certificate:

1. The worker is required to receive pre-employment transition services under Section 113 of the Rehabilitation Act or transition services under the Individuals with Disabilities Education Act.
2. The worker is required to apply for vocational rehabilitation services at the applicable state agency[14] and the worker has either
   - been found ineligible for services from the state agency; or
   - been found to be eligible for services, developed an individualized plan for employment, pursued services for a reasonable period of time, and closed his or her case.
3. The worker is required to receive information and referrals to other resources that offer employment-related services designed to enable the worker to attain competitive integrated employment, earning at least minimum wage.

These provisions took effect in July 2016. As is the case with other components of employment under SMWs, the WIOA provisions relating to SMWs are enforced by the Wage and Hour Division at DOL.[15]

---

[13] WIOA requires less-intensive informational services for these workers. The services are described in the next question.

[14] Vocational rehabilitation is employment-related services for individuals with disabilities. For more information on federal support of state vocational rehabilitation agencies, see CRS Report R43855, *Rehabilitation Act: Vocational Rehabilitation State Grants*, by Benjamin Collins.

[15] See Wage and Hour Fact Sheet #39H at https://www.dol.gov/whd/regs/compliance/whdfs39h.pdf.

WHAT ONGOING SERVICES MUST ALL WORKERS EMPLOYED UNDER AN SMW CERTIFICATE RECEIVE?

WIOA specifies that workers employed under an SMW certificate must receive informational services and referrals to other resources that offer employment-related services with the objective of competitive integrated employment.[16] Workers may choose to continue to work under an SMW certificate after receiving the required informational services.

These informational services apply to all workers employed under a SMW certificate, regardless of the worker's age or work history. The services must be provided every six months during the first year of employment under a SMW certificate and annually thereafter.

[16] See Section 511(c) of the Rehabilitation Act (29 U.S.C. 794g(c)).

In: Individuals with Disabilities
Editor: Aston Delgado
ISBN: 978-1-53615-030-8

Chapter 6

VOCATIONAL REHABILITATION: ADDITIONAL FEDERAL INFORMATION COULD HELP STATES SERVE EMPLOYERS AND FIND JOBS FOR PEOPLE WITH DISABILITIES*

United States Government Accountability Office

ABBREVIATIONS

ADA	Americans with Disabilities Act of 1990
AJC	American Job Center
CSAVR	Council of State Administrators of Vocational Rehabilitation
DOL	Department of Labor

* This is an edited, reformatted and augmented version of the United States Government Accountability Office, Ranking Member, Committee on Health, Education, Labor, and Pensions, U.S. Senate, Publication No. GAO-18-577, dated September 2018.

Education	Department of Education
IPE	Individualized Plan for Employment
ITSC	Information Technology Support Center
MOU	Memorandum of Understanding
NCSAB	National Council of State Agencies for the Blind
RSA	Rehabilitation Services Administration
VR	Vocational Rehabilitation
WIOA	Workforce Innovation and Opportunity Act

WHY GAO DID THIS STUDY

The VR program, administered by Education and state VR agencies, helps people with disabilities obtain employment. In 2014, WIOA made changes to the VR program, increasing its focus on serving employers, promoting career advancement as part of the broader goal of mainstream employment, and coordinating with other workforce programs. GAO was asked to review the VR program under WIOA.

This chapter examines (1) the steps VR agencies have taken under WIOA to work with employers and place individuals in mainstream employment, and the extent Education has addressed any challenges; (2) how VR agencies have coordinated with other workforce programs and the extent federal agencies have addressed any challenges; and (3) how federal agencies have measured state VR agencies' efforts to serve employers. GAO surveyed all 79 VR agencies (74 responded); conducted three discussion groups with 36 state VR officials and four with 29 employers that worked with VR; interviewed VR and other workforce officials in three states, selected for geographic dispersion, among other factors; and reviewed relevant federal laws, regulations, and guidance.

WHAT GAO RECOMMENDS

GAO is making seven recommendations, including improving information on career advancement and partnerships, and aligning performance measures with activities. DOL agreed, while Education neither agreed nor disagreed with the recommendations, but said it will consider taking steps in response.

WHAT GAO FOUND

State vocational rehabilitation (VR) agencies reported expanding services for employers in order to promote hiring individuals with disabilities in mainstream employment (where they are integrated with employees without disabilities and earn competitive wages), but the Department of Education (Education) has not fully addressed related challenges. Most VR agencies in GAO's survey reported providing specific employer services under the Workforce Innovation and Opportunity Act (WIOA) (see figure). However, many agencies reported challenges meeting employers' needs and promoting mainstream employment. For example, some did not fully understand when they are allowed to help employed individuals with career advancement. Education has provided related guidance, including disseminating information at conferences. However, officials at two of three VR agencies GAO spoke with said more information would be helpful. Increasing access to this information may help more VR agencies understand when they have the option of using VR funds for such services.

Most VR agencies GAO surveyed reported increasing coordination with other workforce agencies, but some gaps exist in federal guidance intended to enhance coordination. Employers GAO spoke with cited challenges navigating workforce programs, yet few agencies reported documenting roles and responsibilities of the agencies they partner with to work with employers. While Education and the Department of Labor (DOL) have provided some related technical assistance, they have not provided examples of documentation of roles and responsibilities. GAO's prior work has found that such documentation can help improve coordination by clarifying who does what in a partnership.

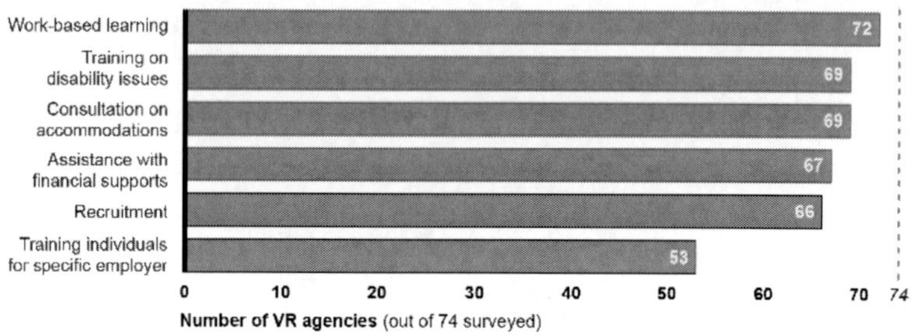

Source: GAO survey of vocational rehabilitation (VR) agencies. | GAO-18-577.

Types of Employer Services Provided by Most State Vocational Rehabilitation Agencies

Education and DOL are piloting three measures of the effectiveness of workforce programs in serving employers: employer penetration (i.e., percentage of employers receiving a service), retention with the same employer, and repeat business customers. However, some VR agencies cited concerns with piloted measures, such as the employer penetration measure not being sufficiently linked to VR core program activities. Taking such concerns into account when finalizing performance measures may result in performance metrics and targets that encourage VR agencies to more effectively serve employers.

* * *

September 6, 2018
The Honorable Patty Murray
Ranking Member
Committee on Health, Education, Labor, and Pensions
United States Senate

Dear Senator Murray:

People with disabilities, including physical, mental, or emotional conditions, often face significant employment challenges. According to the U.S. Bureau of Labor Statistics, in 2016 the average unemployment rate for people with disabilities who are able to work was 10.5 percent, compared to 4.6 percent for those without disabilities.[1] The vocational rehabilitation (VR) program provides services that, among other things, help people with disabilities obtain employment, including counseling and training. In fiscal year 2017, federal funding for the VR program was over $3 billion. The Department of Education (Education) oversees this funding and generally distributes it as grants to the state agencies that administer the VR program.

Studies have found that some employers are reluctant to hire people with disabilities, due, for example, to their perceptions about the costs of accommodations or the work capacity of people with disabilities. Studies have also found that many individuals with significant disabilities have been employed in sheltered workshops, where they are segregated from other employees and may be paid less than minimum wage.[2] The Workforce Innovation and Opportunity Act (WIOA), enacted in 2014, made changes to a range of workforce programs, including changes to the VR program that promote mainstream employment for people with disabilities.[3] For example, WIOA authorized state VR agencies to provide services to employers such as outreach and technical assistance; emphasized the goal of placing VR clients in mainstream employment, where they have competitive wages and are integrated with employees without disabilities; and required Education and the Department of Labor (DOL) to develop one or more performance measures assessing how well VR and certain other workforce programs serve

---

[1] The survey used to determine these unemployment rates defines disability as being deaf, being blind, or having difficulty with various tasks due to a physical, mental, or emotional condition.

[2] According to one recent study, many people in sheltered workshops—center-based, group work settings for people with significant disabilities—are paid sub-minimum wage. According to this study, as of 2016 over 200,000 individuals with significant disabilities were paid under minimum wage as authorized by federal law. Advisory Committee on Increasing Competitive Integrated Employment for Individuals with Disabilities, *Final Report* (Sept. 15, 2016).

[3] WIOA set competitive integrated employment as one goal for VR program participants. In this report, we will generally use the term mainstream employment to refer to competitive integrated employment.

employers. WIOA also encourages collaboration between VR and other workforce programs.

You asked us to examine how VR agencies have engaged employers and collaborated with other workforce programs since the enactment of WIOA. This chapter examines (1) the steps VR agencies have taken under WIOA to work with employers and place individuals in mainstream employment, and the extent to which Education has helped them address any challenges; (2) how VR agencies have coordinated with other workforce programs to effectively serve individual clients and employers, and the extent to which federal agencies have addressed any challenges; and (3) the extent to which Education and DOL have measured VR agencies' efforts to serve employers under WIOA.

To address all three objectives, we used the following methodologies. We reviewed relevant federal laws, regulations, and guidance and technical assistance documents. We surveyed all 79 VR agencies across the country and analyzed responses from 74 agencies.[4] We convened discussion groups with VR agency officials at a national conference, and conducted more in-depth interviews with VR and other workforce program officials in three states. We selected the three states for in-depth interviews to obtain a mix with respect to geographic location, the proportion of the state population in urban versus rural areas, and where the VR agency is situated within the state government, among other factors.[5] We convened discussion groups in three states with employers that have worked with the VR program, which we recruited with the help of VR officials.[6] We applied criteria previously identified by GAO, including standards for internal control in the federal government, and key practices for training, effective interagency

---

[4] In presenting our survey results, we refer to number of agencies responding and did not generalize our findings. Nevertheless, because the responding agencies covered a very large proportion of VR agencies, we concluded that the results would not be materially different if the responses from the missing five agencies had also been captured.

[5] The three states selected for in-depth interviews were Alabama, Arizona, and Maryland. See appendix I for more information on how these states were selected.

[6] We held discussion groups with employers in Alabama, California, and Pennsylvania.

collaboration, and performance measurement. For further details on our objectives, scope, and methodology, see appendix I.[7]

We conducted this performance audit from July 2017 to September 2018 in accordance with generally accepted government auditing standards. Those standards require that we plan and perform the audit to obtain sufficient, appropriate evidence to provide a reasonable basis for our findings and conclusions based on our audit objectives. We believe that the evidence obtained provides a reasonable basis for our findings and conclusions based on our audit objectives.

BACKGROUND

The VR program is authorized under the Rehabilitation Act of 1973, as amended.[8] The VR program provides states with allotments of funds, which are determined according to a formula that considers each state's population, average per capita income, the base amount of VR funds from 1978, and other factors. States are required to contribute by generally matching 21.3 percent of the total VR program expenditures (federal plus non-federal); the federal government's share of the total expenditures is generally 78.7 percent.

At the federal level, the VR program is administered by the Rehabilitation Services Administration (RSA), a component of the Office of Special Education and Rehabilitative Services within Education. At the state level, each state has the option of designating a single state agency to serve all VR clients, or designating one agency to serve VR clients who are blind and a separate agency to serve all remaining VR clients. Across the 50 states, the District of Columbia, and five U.S. territories, 33 states or territories opted for a single agency, and 23 states or territories opted for separate

[7] We also obtained and reviewed data from Education on referrals of VR clients from other workforce programs and co-enrollments in other workforce programs. We decided not to report these data because they are self-reported by clients and state VR agencies we spoke with said that clients may not have known who was referring them or what other programs they were enrolled in, thus potentially leading to under-reporting.

[8] See Pub. L. No. 93-112, 87 Stat. 355, codified as amended at 29 U.S.C. § 701 et seq.

agencies. Therefore, in total, there are 79 VR agencies: 33 combined agencies that serve all VR clients, 23 agencies that serve VR clients who are blind, and 23 general agencies that serve VR clients who are not blind.

One goal of the VR program is to maximize opportunities for individuals with disabilities for competitive integrated employment (i.e., mainstream employment). This is generally defined by statute as employment that, among other criteria, (a) pays at least minimum wage, and at least the customary wage paid by the employer for similar work performed by employees without disabilities; (b) is in a location where the employee with a disability interacts with people who do not have disabilities to the same extent as other employees who are in comparable positions; and (c) that presents opportunities for advancement that are similar to those for employees without disabilities who have similar positions.

To be eligible for VR services, an individual must generally (a) have an impairment that constitutes a substantial impediment to employment, (b) be able to benefit in terms of an employment outcome from VR services, and (c) require VR services to prepare for, secure, retain, advance in, or regain employment. If a VR agency determines that it does not have the resources to serve all eligible individuals in a fiscal year, it must develop an order of selection, in which eligible individuals with the most significant disabilities are prioritized for services and other individuals may be placed on a waiting list.

Before providing any services, the VR agency works with the individual to develop a customized Individualized Plan for Employment (IPE), which spells out, among other things, an employment outcome consistent with the general goal of mainstream employment; the services that are needed to achieve the employment outcome; and timeframes for achieving the employment outcome.[9] The services that VR agencies may provide include career counseling; job placement assistance; training, along with supplies or other services to support training; and assistance with job retention. The VR agency closes a client's case when the client achieves an employment

[9] An employment outcome could also be self-employment or supported employment, in which the individual receives services on a temporary basis such as supplementary assessments, a job trainer at the work site, or social skills training to help him or her retain employment.

outcome, or when a determination is made that the client will not achieve the outcome specified in the IPE.

Key Changes under WIOA

Title IV of WIOA made changes to the VR grants program when WIOA was enacted in July 2014. On August 19, 2016, Education promulgated final regulations related to the VR provisions of WIOA, and Education and DOL promulgated final regulations affecting the broader workforce system. The law included several provisions that change how VR agencies are expected to work with employers and coordinate with other workforce programs.[10] Specifically:

Services for Employers

WIOA authorized VR agencies to use VR grant funds to provide several services to employers that have hired or are interested in hiring people with disabilities. These include providing training and technical assistance regarding the employment of people with disabilities, including training on disability awareness and expanded authority for training regarding the requirements of the Americans with Disabilities Act of 1990 (ADA)[11]; working with employers to recruit, train, and provide work-based experiences to people with disabilities; providing consultation regarding workplace accommodations and assistive technology; and facilitating the use of financial supports for hiring and accommodating people with disabilities.[12] Prior to the enactment of WIOA, VR agencies were authorized to provide a more limited range of services to employers, including

---

[10] WIOA also made other changes affecting the VR program, such as requiring that at least 15 percent of VR funds be used for pre-employment transition services, but our report focuses on changes related to how VR agencies work with employers and other workforce programs.

[11] The ADA provides standards addressing discrimination against individuals with disabilities, and helps ensure that the federal government plays a central role in enforcing these standards, among other things. These standards cover areas such as employment, public services, and public accommodations.

[12] According to an official from the Council of State Administrators of Vocational Rehabilitation (CSAVR), financial supports for hiring people with disabilities include tax incentives.

providing information on compliance with some requirements of the ADA and on VR services.[13]

Job Retention

WIOA provided new flexibility for VR agencies to help individuals retain their jobs, including individuals with less significant disabilities who might not normally be prioritized for services. Under WIOA, when a VR agency is under an order of selection—that is, must prioritize services to certain individuals because the agency lacks the resources to serve all eligible individuals—it may elect to assist individuals who need specific services or equipment to retain employment, even if these individuals would not otherwise receive services under the state's order of selection.

Career Advancement

WIOA put heightened emphasis on helping VR clients advance in their careers in two ways. First, according to Education, WIOA clarified that individuals may qualify for VR services if they need VR services to advance in their careers. Second, WIOA established a definition of competitive integrated employment that includes career advancement opportunities. Prior to the enactment of WIOA, one of the employment outcomes in the VR program was competitive employment in the integrated labor market, but there was no criterion related to advancement opportunities.

Coordination with Other Workforce Programs

WIOA specified that VR is one of six core programs in the workforce system. The other programs are Title I Adult, Title I Dislocated Worker, Title I Youth, Wagner-Peyser Employment Services, and Adult Education and Family Literacy (see app. II for further information). Moreover, for a state to receive allotments under each core program, WIOA requires the governor to submit either a unified state plan or combined state plan for all

---

[13] WIOA authorized VR agencies to provide training and technical assistance on all of the requirements of the ADA related to the employment of individuals with disabilities.

of the core programs.[14] These plans outline a 4-year strategy and describe the workforce needs in the state and how the core programs under WIOA will be administered and aligned or coordinated. For example, one way that the workforce programs may coordinate is by blending or braiding funds —that is, accessing or coordinating multiple sources of funding—which may produce greater strength, efficiency, or effectiveness in support of a common activity or project than the use of any single funding stream.[15]

Measuring Performance in Serving Employers

WIOA required Education and DOL after consultation with state agencies and others[16] to develop and establish one or more performance indicators for "effectiveness in serving employers."[17] These indicators are shared across the six core WIOA programs. For the other five core program performance indicators established by WIOA, the states and the Secretaries of Education and Labor negotiate a combined target performance level for each state, starting from the performance targets included in the unified state plans. The federal agencies have not yet issued guidance on how the target performance level for effectiveness in serving employers will be negotiated.

---

[14] A combined state plan includes the WIOA core programs as well as at least one other partner program, as opposed to the unified state plan, which applies to the core programs only.

[15] U.S. Department of Health and Human Services, Administration for Children and Families, Office of Child Care, *Layering or Blending and Braiding Multiple Funding Streams,* date accessed: May 9, 2018, https://childcareta.acf.hhs.gov/systemsbuilding/systems-guides/financing-strategically/max imizing-impact-public-funding/blending-braiding-funding. In braiding strategies, funding streams remain visible and expenditures are tracked by funding source, whereas with blending, funds are wrapped into a common pool and expenditures are not tracked by funding source. According to Education, blending of funds is constrained by factors including federal guidance that grant funds be used only for allowable program costs.

[16] For example, WIOA requires consultation with representatives of business and industry, employees, and researchers.

[17] WIOA established six primary indicators of performance for the core programs, which are generally as follows: employment rate in the 2nd quarter after exiting the program, employment rate in the 4th quarter after exiting the program, median earnings in the 2nd quarter after exiting the program, credential attainment rate within 1 year of exiting the program, measurable skill gains, and effectiveness in serving employers. Pub. L. No. 113-128, § 116(b), 128 Stat. 1425, 1471.

Workforce System

Under federal law—both before and after enactment of WIOA—states and local areas are required to bring together a number of federally funded employment and training programs into a comprehensive network of partners, now called the American Job Center (AJC) network. An AJC is a physical location where clients—including job seekers with and without disabilities and employers seeking employees—can access the programs, services, and activities of the various workforce partners. States also must establish workforce development boards at the state and local levels. At the state-level, these boards are responsible for assisting the governor in developing and improving the statewide workforce system, and at the local level, they are responsible for serving as the strategic leader and convener of local workforce system stakeholders. WIOA requires the local board to develop and enter into a Memorandum of Understanding (MOU) between the local board and the workforce programs at the AJC concerning the operation of the AJC delivery system in a local area.

Guidance and Technical Assistance

DOL's Employment and Training Administration— the entity within DOL responsible for providing national oversight of the workforce investment system—and Education's RSA and Office of Career, Technical, and Adult Education have provided various types of guidance and technical assistance to state agencies to help implement WIOA. After WIOA increased the emphasis on services for employers and collaboration across the workforce development system, Education and DOL issued technical assistance circulars and joint guidance on these priorities. Education and DOL also provide technical assistance directly to state agencies through conference presentations, regional meetings, webinars, and websites.

In addition, Education conducts annual reviews and periodic on-site monitoring of state VR programs. Education also created several grant-funded technical assistance centers to help VR agencies implement WIOA.

These technical assistance centers are largely staffed by academics and provide a range of assistance such as conference presentations, newsletters, and more intensive assistance to individual states. In particular, one of the technical assistance centers—the Job-Driven Vocational Rehabilitation Technical Assistance Center—focuses on providing assistance related to employer engagement and employer supports. Another technical assistance center—the Workforce Innovation Technical Assistance Center—provides assistance focused on helping integrate VR into the workforce system.

AbilityOne Program

Under the AbilityOne program, people who are blind or have other severe disabilities are employed to provide products and services to federal agencies.[18] The program typically provides products such as office supplies and military apparel, and services such as janitorial, landscaping, and document destruction. Federal agencies that need the products and services on the AbilityOne Program Procurement List are required to buy them from AbilityOne authorized nonprofit agencies employing people who are blind or have severe disabilities. The AbilityOne program is administered by the U.S. AbilityOne Commission, which oversees a network of nonprofit agencies. The U.S. AbilityOne Commission establishes program rules and regulations, determines what products and services the program provides, and sets prices for these products and services.

The U.S. AbilityOne Commission authorized two central nonprofit agencies—SourceAmerica and National Industries for the Blind—to facilitate the distribution, by direct allocation, subcontract, or any other means, of orders of the federal government for products and services on the procurement list among qualified nonprofit agencies. By statute, the program requires that at least 75 percent of a nonprofit agency's total direct labor hours during the fiscal year be carried out by people who are blind or have severe disabilities. As of 2018, over 500 nonprofit agencies across the

[18] See 41 U.S.C. § 8501 et seq.

country participate in the AbilityOne program and train and employ people with disabilities to provide products and services to federal agencies. According to data provided by the U.S. AbilityOne Commission, in fiscal year 2016 the program employed 46,161 people.

VR Agencies Have Reported Expanding Employer Services, but Education Has Not Fully Addressed Challenges Related to Employer Needs and Mainstream Employment

Most VR Agencies Reported Enhancing a Range of Employer Services

Most state VR agencies reported in our survey that they have enhanced their services for employers under WIOA. Fifty of the 74 agencies that responded to our survey reported they have enhanced services in some way, including 36 that increased both the overall level of services to employers and provided services in a more formal, well-defined way; 11 that increased the overall level of services; and 3 that provided services in a more formal, well-defined way. Also, most VR agencies (61 of 74) reported that they have staff members dedicated to working with employers, and about a third of these agencies (22 of 61) reported that they increased the number of staff dedicated to serving employers under WIOA. Survey responses also revealed that fewer VR agencies that serve only people who are blind or visually impaired (12 of 21, or 57 percent) have staff dedicated to working with employers, compared to VR agencies that only serve the general disability population (22 of 23, or 96 percent) or those that serve all VR clients (27 of 30, or 90 percent). Officials from the National Council of State Agencies for the Blind (NCSAB) told us that due to their small size, VR agencies serving the blind population often have staff perform multiple functions and therefore typically do not have staff who specialize in working with employers. When asked whether agencies for the blind therefore face challenges in working with employers, NCSAB officials said that VR agencies for the blind may coordinate with general VR agencies on employer engagement, and that more agencies for the blind are developing their own employer specialists.

VR agency officials we spoke with in discussion groups and interviews echoed our survey results, indicating they are either taking substantial new steps to work with employers, or expanding services that they were already providing. For example, a VR official in one discussion group said that they have historically focused on serving individual clients with disabilities, and are now trying to develop expertise in serving employers as well. Meanwhile, officials at one VR agency that has worked with employers for many years told us that they expanded the number of staff who focus on working with employers from one to eight, and are putting more emphasis on educating employers about the ADA and reasonable accommodations, which they see as a priority area in WIOA.[19]

In addition to reporting that they enhanced employer services, the majority of VR agencies reported in our survey that they provide various employer services authorized by WIOA (see fig.1).[20]

VR agency officials we spoke with cited several specific aspects of how they work with employers as being especially effective:

- VR agency officials in two of our three discussion groups said that establishing a relationship with an employer is important, and officials in one discussion group said that this is important

---

[19] The ADA generally requires an employer to provide reasonable accommodations to an employee or job applicant with a disability, unless doing so would cause undue hardship. According to the Equal Employment Opportunity Commission, in general, a reasonable accommodation is any change in the work environment that helps a person with a disability apply for or perform a job. This could include, for example, making a workplace wheelchair accessible or providing an interpreter for someone who is hearing impaired.

[20] Our findings are consistent with those of another survey conducted shortly after the enactment of WIOA. That survey found that 59 of 66 responding VR agencies served employers as customers, and the top five most commonly provided services for employers included accommodations, training on disability issues, assistance with financial supports, and recruitment. Kelly Haines, et al., *Vocational Rehabilitation and Business Relations: Preliminary Indicators of State VR Agency Capacity*, Journal of Vocational Rehabilitation 48 (2018).

specifically so that employers will contact the VR agency when an employee needs help with keeping his or her job.

- Officials we interviewed in another VR agency said that work-based learning such as apprenticeships is especially useful in connecting employers and people with disabilities, because it provides on-the-job experience and is often in in-demand occupations.
- And in one of our discussion groups, an official from a different VR agency said that it is valuable to understand an employer's specific skill needs and pre-screen job candidates before referring them to ensure a good match.

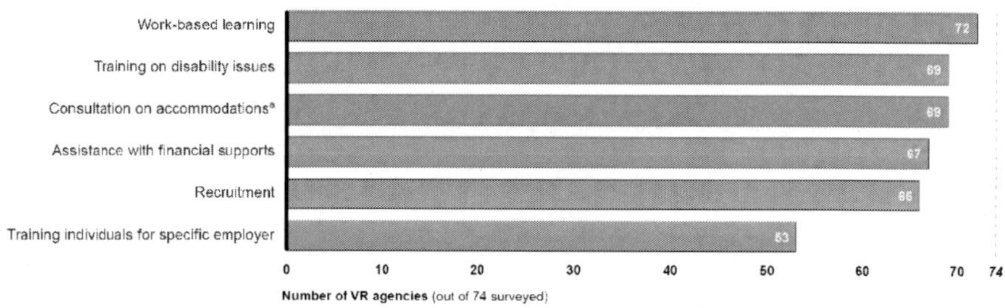

Source: GAO survey of vocational rehabilitation (VR) agencies. | GAO-18-577.

Note: The survey question was: "Does your agency currently provide any of the following services to employers either formally (e.g., as a distinct or well-defined program) or informally (e.g., by individual counselors in the course of their routine duties)?" Seventy-four VR agencies answered this question.

[a] According to the Equal Employment Opportunity Commission, a reasonable accommodation, in general, is any change in the work environment that helps a person with a disability apply for or perform a job.

Figure 1. Number of State VR Agencies that Reported Providing Selected Services Authorized by the Workforce Innovation and Opportunity Act to Employers.

Employers we spoke with echoed these comments about how VR services are useful. For example, employers in two of four discussion groups said that VR agencies' efforts to maintain relationships have been helpful, employers in two discussion groups emphasized the value of receiving pre-screened job candidates from VR agencies, and employers in one discussion group said that paid work experience—in which VR pays a portion of an employee's wages for a period of time—has been a helpful and low-cost way to try out a job candidate with disabilities.

In addition to the above services to employers, almost all VR agencies (72 of 74) reported that they help employers keep their employees by providing job retention assistance to individuals with disabilities. Fewer agencies reported that they are acting on new flexibility under WIOA to provide job retention services to individuals who would not otherwise qualify under the state's order of selection. (As noted previously, a VR agency develops an order of selection, which prioritizes services to individuals with the most significant disabilities, when it lacks resources to serve all eligible individuals.) Specifically, of the 30 VR agencies that reported being on an order of selection at the time of our survey, about half (14) reported that they have elected to provide job retention services to individuals who would not otherwise be prioritized for VR services under the order of selection. Officials we interviewed at one VR agency said that they opted not to provide job retention services to individuals outside their order of selection because of the need to prioritize services to people with the most significant disabilities.

VR Agencies Reported Challenges with Meeting Employer Needs and Promoting Mainstream Employment, Which Education Has Not Fully Addressed

VR agencies we surveyed and interviewed, and employers we interviewed said that they have experienced several challenges, such as those related to VR agencies' training for employers, ability to quickly meet employers' needs (i.e., working at the speed of business), and marketing. Other challenges are related to VR agencies' ability to promote mainstream employment for their clients, including in the area of career advancement. However, Education has not consistently addressed these challenges through the information and assistance it provides.

Training for Employers

Employers expressed concerns about the in-person format VR agencies use to provide training on disability issues. Employers in three of four discussion groups said that it can be difficult to get front-line supervisors together at one time to attend in-person trainings offered by VR agencies, and it would be helpful to have more flexible, on-demand training options. For example, several employers in one discussion group said that it would be useful to have online training options that their front-line managers can take individually at their convenience. Similarly, employers in another discussion group said it is hard to schedule training each time a new person enters a supervisory position, so it would be useful to have on-demand options such as pre-recorded videos. Officials we interviewed at the three VR agencies told us that they do not provide on-demand or online trainings for employers. An official at one of these agencies said that they provide only in-person trainings because they believe this format is more effective in building a relationship with the employer and promoting the hiring of people with disabilities.

While Education has provided technical assistance to VR agencies on training employers, it does not provide assistance related to the format of this training. Officials from the Job-Driven Vocational Rehabilitation Technical Assistance Center told us that the center has provided intensive technical assistance to VR agencies on the importance of educating employers about hiring and working with people with disabilities. This center also offers VR agencies information on disability awareness and the ADA to help VR agencies educate employers about these issues. However, while the center has posted some videos on its website that discus VR success stories in working with employers, center officials said that they have not developed online training or multimedia presentations for employers. Education officials said that while they see potential value in on-demand and online training for some employers, they have not directed the technical assistance centers to provide assistance to VR agencies on using these training formats because they have not heard about this issue from VR agencies or employers.[21]

We have previously reported that agencies should consider providing trainees with the flexibility to choose among different training delivery methods (such as web-based and instructor-led) while leveraging resources in the most efficient way possible.[22] Further, standards for internal control in the federal government state that federal agency management should communicate quality information so that external parties, including other government entities, can help the entity achieve its objectives and address related risks.[23] VR agencies are authorized to provide training to employers on disability issues, which is one way to achieve one of the program's objectives of promoting employment for people with disabilities. By providing information to VR agencies on how to deliver training to employers in formats, such as on-demand videos, that best meet employers' needs, Education, through its technical assistance centers, may improve VR agencies' ability to customize training for individual employers, reach a broader range of front-line supervisors, and thereby better achieve program objectives. While in-person training may help with developing relationships with employers, alternative training formats such as on-demand videos could supplement—not replace—in-person training. Moreover, VR agency officials we interviewed also mentioned other ways to cultivate such relationships, such as regular communication with employers that may include sharing articles on disability issues, or providing services an employer needs such as accessibility assessments.

Working at the Speed of Business

VR agency officials and employers said that VR agencies sometimes face challenges meeting employers' hiring and other needs in a timely

---

[21] Education also said that information for employers on hiring people with disabilities is available from other sources—such as the Americans with Disabilities Act Knowledge Translation Center—in alternative formats that include videos.

[22] GAO, *Human Capital: A Guide for Assessing Strategic Training and Development Efforts in the Federal Government*, GAO-04-546G (Washington, D.C.: March 2004).

[23] GAO, *Standards for Internal Control in the Federal Government*, GAO-14-704G (Washington, D.C.: September 2014).

manner. On our survey, 45 of 74 VR agencies reported that quickly meeting employers' needs is moderately, very, or extremely difficult.[24] Similarly, VR agency officials in one of three discussion groups said that it can be challenging meeting employers' needs given the agency's limited resources, citing, for example, the extensive staff time required to evaluate an employment site's accessibility. Officials we interviewed at one VR agency also noted that it can be difficult to meet employers' immediate need for a certain number of qualified job candidates, due, for example, to the time it takes to prepare VR clients for specific jobs. Employers expressed similar concerns. Employers in one of four discussion groups said that VR does not always provide enough qualified job candidates to meet their needs, and employers in another discussion group said that job candidates referred by VR are not always good matches for their hiring needs.

Officials at Education's technical assistance centers said that they have provided information and technical assistance to VR agencies to help them address these challenges. For example, they have worked with VR agencies on developing new approaches to engaging employers, with a focus on understanding employers' needs and coordinating within the VR agency to quickly refer job candidates that meet these needs, if such are available. They have also provided documents with examples of how VR agencies can collaborate with employers, such as "What is Business Engagement?," which identifies sectors of the economy with high demand for workers and describes strategies for building relationships with employers and meeting their needs. Technical assistance officials said that the centers have also facilitated sharing of promising practices among VR agencies and encouraged VR agencies to use an online tool designed to connect employers with job seekers with disabilities. Officials we interviewed at the three VR agencies said that they have used or plan to use the online recruitment tool, and one also commented that sharing of best practices among the states has been helpful.

---

[24] The survey asked about difficulty with "meeting the demands of businesses (e.g., speed of services to businesses, fitting into the work schedules of businesses)."

Outreach to Employers

VR agencies and employers cited challenges with ensuring employers are aware of the services available from the VR program. Thirty-one of the 74 VR agencies that responded to our survey reported that marketing VR services to employers is moderately, very, or extremely difficult, and VR agency officials in two of three discussion groups said that marketing and awareness of VR among employers is a challenge. Officials we interviewed in all three VR agencies provided examples of challenges related to outreach, such as limited resources to conduct outreach, reluctance on the part of some employers to hire people with disabilities, and turnover among VR staff which makes it difficult to maintain relationships with employers. At the same time, employers in three of four discussion groups said that VR agencies need to do more marketing to get the word out about their services.

Representatives from the Job-Driven Vocational Rehabilitation Technical Assistance Center have taken several steps to help VR agencies inform employers about their services. Among other things, they provided a toolkit with resources that VR agencies can draw on when developing their outreach efforts, including information on using social media in marketing; and established a marketing affinity group to help VR agencies share tips and ideas and form cross-state partnerships. Officials we interviewed from two VR agencies either told us they have found the outreach materials provided by the technical assistance centers useful or did not indicate the need for any additional assistance in this area.

Career Advancement

VR agencies and employers cited issues with implementing WIOA's heightened emphasis on career advancement for VR clients. VR agency officials in two of three discussion groups said that it has been a cultural shift for VR staff to focus on career advancement, and not solely on job placement. In our survey, 41 of 74 VR agencies reported that it was moderately, very, or extremely difficult to find jobs in which employees with disabilities have similar advancement opportunities as those without disabilities, which is a goal established by WIOA. In addition, some VR agencies have been reluctant to provide career advancement services to VR clients who are already employed, which could include training for an advanced degree. For example, officials we interviewed at one VR agency said there is some confusion about whether VR clients who are employed can qualify for additional VR services for advancement. They explained that, under the statutory eligibility criteria, an individual's disability must constitute a substantial impediment to employment—and some agency officials believe that someone who is already employed cannot have a disability that is a substantial impediment to employment. Officials we interviewed at the other two VR agencies said that their agencies typically do not provide advancement services to people who are employed because their resources are limited, and they prioritize services to people who are not yet employed. Meanwhile, employers in two of four discussion groups said that they would like more assistance from VR agencies with promoting career advancement for their employees with disabilities, and employers in one of the other two groups were not aware that VR could provide such assistance.[25]

Education and one of its technical assistance centers have provided information to states on how to promote career advancement. Officials from the Workforce Innovation Technical Assistance Center said that they have provided intensive assistance to states on The Career Index Plus, an online career information system.[26] They also have provided assistance on developing career pathways that combine training and work experience, including for people with disabilities. Furthermore, Education officials said that they provided information to VR agencies at three conferences from November 2017 to March 2018, to address states' needs for clarification about when VR clients may be provided career advancement services. In their presentations, Education officials explained that the VR program is intended to help individuals achieve employment that is appropriate for their skills and preferences, and is not limited to just entry-level jobs; that VR

[25] In our fourth employer discussion group, one employer said it would be helpful for the VR program to provide more assistance with career advancement, but this opinion did not emerge as a consistent theme across multiple discussion group participants.

[26] According to technical assistance center officials, The Career Index Plus includes information on careers such as job projections, licenses and certification requirements, and related occupations for career advancement planning.

services may include graduate level education if needed for advancement in a current job or into a new job; and that an individual's employment and education should not be factors in determining VR eligibility.

However, Education may not have fully addressed states' information needs. Officials we interviewed from two of three VR agencies told us between December 2017 and March 2018 that additional information on providing career advancement services to employed individuals would be helpful. Furthermore, one respondent to our survey wrote that many states are unable to attend conferences, and suggested that information should be disseminated more widely. Education officials said that they were not aware of widespread confusion among VR agencies or the need for more assistance on these issues, and therefore had no plans to disseminate further information. Education officials also acknowledged that they were not aware that some VR agencies have opted not to serve employed individuals because they are on an order of selection.

Standards for internal control in the federal government state that federal agency management should communicate quality information to external parties including government entities, such as through written documents or meetings, so that these parties can help the entity achieve its objectives and address related risks.[27] One aspect of providing quality information is ensuring that this information is accessible. While promoting career advancement for individuals with disabilities is emphasized by WIOA, our review suggests that VR agencies may lack sufficient access to information on the circumstances in which they can provide advancement services to employed individuals with disabilities, including when resources are constrained. In turn, VR agencies may not realize they have the option to assist this population in developing their full career potential.

AbilityOne Program

VR agencies have historically been a significant source of referrals to the nonprofit agencies that operate the AbilityOne program, according to officials from the U.S. AbilityOne Commission. However, WIOA

---

[27] GAO-14-704G.

emphasizes mainstream employment and Education's regulations and guidance under WIOA provide further details about how VR agencies may refer clients to AbilityOne jobs. While federal law states that VR participants should exercise informed choice over their individual employment goals, WIOA specifies that mainstream—i.e., competitive and integrated—employment is a goal of the VR program.[28] Education's regulations implementing WIOA further specify that with respect to an employment outcome, an integrated setting is generally one typically found in the community, and where individuals with disabilities interact with other employees without disabilities "within the particular work unit" to the same extent that comparable employees without disabilities do. In its responses to frequently asked questions, Education further explains that a work unit may refer to all employees in a particular job category or to a group of employees working together to accomplish tasks.

In guidance to state VR agencies, Education also provides some direction as to how VR agencies should apply this criterion. In the preamble to its VR regulations, as well as in responses to frequently asked questions, Education emphasizes that VR agencies must apply this regulatory criterion to each employment setting on a case-by-case basis to determine if it qualifies as integrated. However, the preamble and Education's responses to frequently asked questions also state that jobs supported by the AbilityOne program generally do not meet the criterion of being typically found in the community, and therefore generally do not qualify as integrated settings.

Some stakeholders told us the AbilityOne program can provide integrated settings for some people with disabilities, while others expressed concerns that the program generally does not promote mainstream employment. Officials from the U.S. AbilityOne Commission told us that certain AbilityOne positions—especially service jobs such as janitorial—can offer a setting where people with disabilities are integrated with people who do not have disabilities. For example, janitors in a federal building

---

[28] Under federal law, VR participants are to be active and full participants in the VR process, making meaningful and informed choices over, among other things, the selection of employment outcomes for the individuals, services needed to achieve the outcomes, entities providing such services, and the methods used to secure such services.

working under an AbilityOne contract might be spread out across the building, working alongside other building staff without disabilities. In contrast, a report by the Advisory Committee on Increasing Competitive Integrated Employment for Individuals with Disabilities states that the AbilityOne program is not consistent with the goal of increasing mainstream employment, and recommended that Congress amend the AbilityOne program's authorizing statute to promote greater integration of people with disabilities into mainstream employment settings. Furthermore, representatives we interviewed from two disability organizations said that there is general support in the disability community for moving away from the types of segregated work settings often provided through AblIltyOne and toward more mainstream employment.

Many VR agencies have reduced their referrals of clients to the nonprofit agencies participating in the AbilityOne program since the enactment of WIOA, according to our survey; and a number of state VR officials told us in interviews and discussion groups that in their view Education's regulations or guidance indicate that AbilityOne jobs should not be seen as mainstream employment. At a national level, 31 of 74 VR agencies responding to our survey reported that they have either decreased or completely ceased referrals to the AbilityOne program under WIOA (see fig. 2).[29] Officials we interviewed at three VR agencies said they are less likely to actively refer clients to AbilityOne because there is uncertainty about whether it qualifies as mainstream employment, which affects whether it can be considered a successful employment outcome under WIOA. Officials in two of these three states—as well as state VR agency officials in all three of our discussion groups—noted their view that Education's regulations or guidance discourage them from treating AbilityOne jobs as mainstream employment. For example, VR officials we interviewed in one

[29] The survey question was: "Since the passage of WIOA, is your agency more or less likely to refer clients to AbilityOne positions?" Our survey did not ask why VR agencies may have changed their rate of referrals to AbilityOne. Therefore, we cannot infer from the survey responses whether (a) VR agencies are assessing AbilityOne jobs on a case-by-case basis to determine if they are integrated, as called for by Education's guidance; or (b) VR agencies are—consistent with federal law—referring clients to AbilityOne jobs when that is their choice, even if the VR agency does not consider the job to be mainstream employment.

state said that, in their view, AbilityOne jobs do not qualify as mainstream. They explained that while employees with disabilities in these jobs may interact with employees without disabilities who are doing other types of work at the same work site, they tend to be in work crews or settings where they work directly only with other employees with disabilities. They said this is not consistent with the work unit provision in the regulations, which they interpret as requiring that for a work setting to qualify as integrated, employees with disabilities must work directly with and do the exact same type of work as employees without disabilities. At the same time, officials we interviewed at all three state VR agencies said that they do not dissuade VR clients from entering the AbilityOne program, if that is their choice.

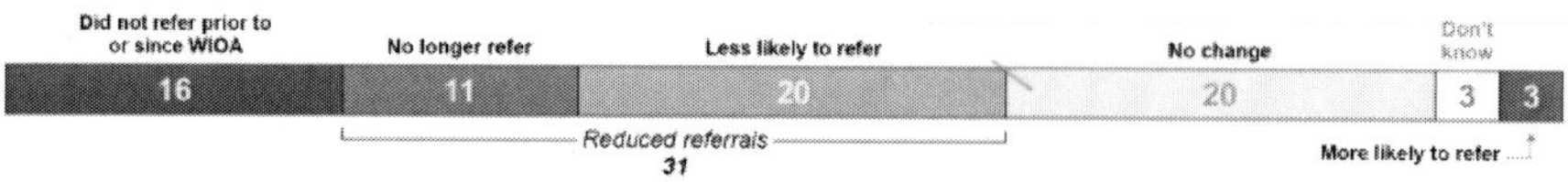

Source: GAO survey of voational rehabiitation (VR) agencies. | GAO-18-577.

WIOA= Workforce Innovation and Opportunity Act.

Note: The survey question was: "Since the passage of WIOA, is your agency more or less likely to refer clients to AbilityOne positions?" Seventy-three agencies answered this question. Our survey did not ask why VR agencies may have changed their rate of referrals to AbilityOne. Therefore, we cannot infer from the survey responses whether (a) VR agencies are assessing AbilityOne jobs on a case-by-case basis to determine if they are integrated, as called for by Education's guidance; or (b) VR agencies are—consistent with federal law—referring clients to AbilityOne jobs when that is their choice, even if the VR agency does not consider the job to be mainstream employment.

Figure 2. Number of VR Agencies That Have Changed Their Referrals to AbilityOne Authorized Nonprofit Agencies under WIOA.

Our survey and discussion groups with state VR agencies indicate that agencies struggle to find good jobs outside of AbilityOne for some individuals. In our survey, 33 of 74 VR agencies reported that it was moderately, very, or extremely difficult to find jobs in integrated settings—an aspect of mainstream employment—for clients who would otherwise be good candidates for AbilityOne. Among this group, more than half of the agencies serving the blind population (12 of 21, or 57 percent) reported that this was moderately to extremely challenging, compared to smaller proportions of general agencies (8 of 23, or 35 percent) and combined agencies (13 of 30, or 43 percent). Officials from NCSAB told us that many blind VR customers have chosen to work in AbilityOne settings because these individuals tend to face challenges with discrimination or inaccessible software in the mainstream labor market. In addition, officials in two of three discussion groups said the reduction in referrals to AbilityOne has been challenging because AbilityOne jobs often pay good wages.[30] For example, one official said that the VR agency now places clients in jobs where they are more integrated with people without disabilities but earn less.

While a number of VR agencies told us that they have reduced their referrals to the AbilityOne program as a result of Education's regulations and guidance, our discussion groups and interviews with officials also suggest that VR agencies may have interpreted Education's guidance related to the case-by-case review in different ways. On one hand, VR agency officials in two of three discussion groups told us that they assess AbilityOne employment settings on a case-by-case basis to determine if they qualify as mainstream employment under WIOA and Education's regulations. Officials we interviewed at one VR agency told us that some AbilityOne positions qualify as mainstream employment. On the other hand, VR officials representing several agencies told us—either in discussion groups or in our interviews—that Education's regulations or guidance preclude AbilityOne from qualifying as mainstream employment or that the guidance is not clear on the matter. Also, VR agency officials in one of our three discussion groups said that given their limited resources, it is difficult to assess each AbilityOne position to determine if it qualifies as integrated.

Education officials said that when they have become aware of VR agencies deciding that no AbilityOne jobs qualify as mainstream employment, they provided technical assistance to these agencies about the

---

[30] According to data provided by the U.S. AbilityOne Commission, during fiscal year 2016 the average wage for AbilityOne positions managed by National Industries for the Blind was $11.17 per hour, and the average wage for AbilityOne positions managed by SourceAmerica was $13.28 per hour. U.S. AbilityOne Commission officials also said that some individuals in AbilityOne jobs are paid sub-minimum wages as authorized by federal law, but that data on this number were not available.

need to assess these jobs on a case-by-case basis. Education officials said that they are reviewing the agency's regulations and non-regulatory guidance overall in response to an executive order, but otherwise had no specific plans to provide additional or clarifying information to VR agencies.[31]

Standards for internal control in the federal government state that federal agency management should communicate quality information so that external parties can help the entity achieve its objectives and address related risks.[32] One aspect of providing quality information is ensuring that it is complete. The fact that state VR agencies said they have different interpretations of the information provided by Education on integrated employment settings suggests this information may not be sufficiently complete or high-quality. Without more complete information from Education on whether or how to assess AbilityOne jobs to determine if they qualify as integrated, VR agencies may continue to interpret the information provided by Education in different ways, which could potentially undermine the program's mission of placing individuals with disabilities in mainstream employment.

VR Agencies Have Increased Coordination, but Federal Agencies Have Not Fully Addressed Challenges Related to Clarifying Roles and Data Sharing

Many VR Agencies Reported Increased Coordination under WIOA

Most VR agencies reported in our survey that they have increased their overall level of coordination with workforce partners—to serve both

---

[31] Executive Order 13777, issued on February 24, 2017, requires each agency to set up a Regulatory Reform Task Force to review its existing regulations and make recommendations for their repeal, modification, or replacement.

[32] GAO-14-704G.

individuals and employers—under WIOA. Sixty-nine of the 74 VR agencies that responded to our survey reported that their overall level of coordination has increased since the enactment of WIOA; specifically, 61 increased both the overall level of coordination and conducted that coordination in a more formal, well-defined way; 7 increased the overall level of coordination but did not increase the formality of the coordination; and 1 increased the overall level of coordination but reduced the formality of it.[33]

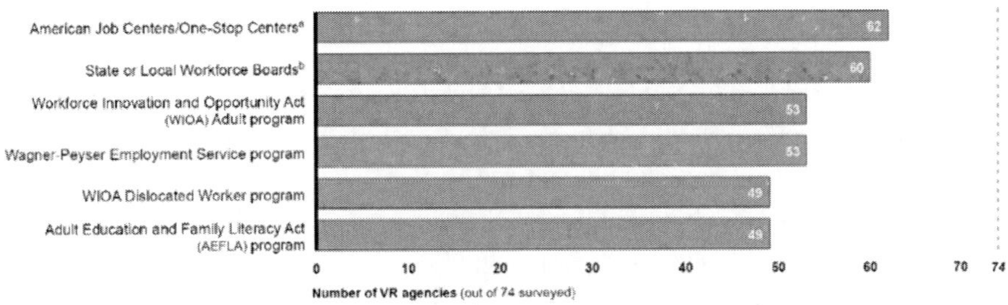

Source: GAO survey of vocational rehabilitation (VR) agencies. | GAO-18-577.

Notes: The survey question was: "Which of the following workforce partners does your agency currently coordinate with...in order to help VR clients obtain or maintain employment? This coordination could be done as part of a formal, well-defined program or informally, e.g., by individual counselors as the need arises." The number of agencies that responded for each sub-question was: American Job Centers (73); State or Local Workforce Boards (73); WIOA Adult program (72); Wagner-Peyser Employment Service program (72); WIOA Dislocated Worker program (71); AEFLA Program (73).

[a] American Job Centers (AJCs) are the physical locations where clients can access the programs, services, and activities of the various workforce partners. They were formerly called One-Stop Centers and re-branded as AJCs in 2016.

[b] States must establish workforce development boards at the state and local levels. At the state-level, these boards are responsible for assisting the governor in developing and improving the statewide workforce system, and at the local level, they are responsible for serving as the strategic leader and convener of local workforce system stakeholders.

Figure 3. Number of State VR Agencies That Reported Coordinating with Other Workforce Programs and Entities.

[33] However, the state did not provide comments on how they increased the level of coordination while reducing the formality of it.

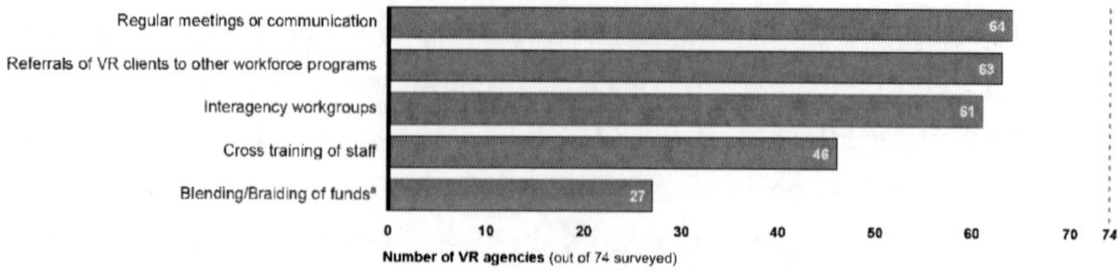

Source: GAO survey of vocational rehabilitation (VR) agencies. | GAO-18-577.

Notes: The survey question was: "In which of the following ways does your agency currently coordinate with other workforce partners (such as American Job Centers/One-Stop Centers, State or local workforce boards, WIOA Adult, WIOA Dislocated Worker, Wagner-Peyser Employment Service Program) on engaging with employers and/or helping clients obtain and retain employment? This coordination could be done as part of a formal, well-defined program or informally, e.g., by individual counselors as the need arises." The number of agencies that responded for each sub-question was: Regular meetings or communication (73); Cross referrals (74); Interagency workgroups (73); Cross training of staff (74); Blending/Braiding of funds (71).

[a] One way that the workforce programs may coordinate is by blending or braiding funds—that is, accessing or coordinating multiple sources of funding—which may produce greater strength, efficiency, or effectiveness in support of a common activity or project than the use of any single funding stream.

Figure 4. Number of State VR Agencies That Reported Conducting Various Coordination Activities.

In all three states with which we conducted in-depth interviews, state VR agencies and labor officials described overall enhanced coordination under WIOA, reflecting greater integration of VR into the workforce system. One state VR agency official explained that WIOA has pushed VR agencies to think more about what the other workforce programs are doing and how VR services can be integrated with them, resulting in, for example, a successful joint labor-VR career fair for people with disabilities. Another state VR official noted her state conducted 12 different sets of negotiations to develop an MOU. Through that process, the agencies have developed a better understanding of their partners' needs and what services they might be able to take advantage of.

Most VR agencies reported in our survey that they coordinate with various workforce programs and entities under WIOA, most frequently with AJCs and workforce boards (see fig. 3).

In our survey, VR agencies also reported coordinating with workforce programs through regular communication, interagency workgroups, cross referrals and, to a lesser extent, cross-training and blending/braiding of funds (see fig. 4). Based on our review, we determined that these coordination practices being carried out by workforce programs are consistent with best practices previously identified by GAO—practices that include bridging organizational culture, identifying participants, and identifying resources to support the interagency collaboration.[34]

In our in-depth interviews, VR and other state officials provided additional details about these reported activities, as follows:

- *Regular meetings or communication* - One state VR agency official we interviewed said that the agency holds mandatory monthly meetings to collaborate across programs on working with employers.
- *Cross referrals* - In one state, VR staff told us that there are a couple of cross referrals between the workforce programs per week. For example, AJC staff send individuals with disabilities to VR staff, and VR staff meet with those individuals in the AJC office.
- *Interagency workgroups* - At one AJC, officials said that they use task forces or workgroups that bring together workforce programs and other entities, such as nonprofits and staffing agencies, to discuss client needs, skills, and job availability. Having such interagency communication helps ensure that participants are included and engaged in the interagency collaboration.

---

[34] GAO, Managing for Results: Key Considerations for Implementing Interagency Collaborative Mechanisms, GAO-12-1022 (Washington, D.C.: September 2012). The key features of interagency collaboration include outcomes and accountability, bridging organizational culture, leadership, clarity of roles and responsibilities, participants, resources, and written guidance and agreements. We describe in this section how each of these practices is or is not reflected in the coordination we found across workforce programs, except outcomes and accountability, which is described in the next section.

- *Cross training staff* - VR agency officials in one state said that their state has held quarterly trainings for all employer relations staff at different workforce development agencies, which included information on disability issues such as the ADA and appropriate ways for employers to interact with employees with disabilities. These officials noted that this training has helped employer relations staff from other programs at the AJCs conduct outreach to employers regarding disability issues and hiring people with disabilities. Cross training can enable agencies to bridge organizational culture, because they become familiar with the terminology and services of other programs.[35]
- *Leveraging multiple funding streams to serve clients* - While fewer states reported leveraging multiple funding streams in our survey than other coordination activities, all three of the states where we conducted in-depth interviews reported doing so. For example, in one state, a VR agency official told us about a program in which her agency placed clients in internships, while the clients received a living stipend from a state department of labor grant program. When asked why multiple funding streams were not leveraged more, one official said that their state has been focused on implementing the mandatory provisions of WIOA up until this point; another official noted that it is better to keep funds separate and helpful to have funds designated for people with disabilities rather than mixing funds.

Few VR Agencies Reported Documenting Clear Roles and Sharing Data, and Gaps Exist in Federal Assistance

Documenting Roles and Responsibilities

Few state VR agencies reported documenting roles and responsibilities among workforce program staff with respect to working with employers,

[35] GAO-12-1022.

which may have contributed to challenges with serving employers. Establishing and documenting clear roles and responsibilities is a key consideration for implementing collaboration mechanisms, according to prior GAO work.[36] In our survey, fewer than half of VR agencies (28 of 73) reported establishing clear roles and responsibilities for VR staff and for the other workforce program staff with respect to working with employers.[37] Only 15 of 73 state VR agencies reported that they had written documentation of those roles. Forty-one of 73 state VR agencies reported that documenting clear roles and responsibilities is a work in progress.

We also found that several local MOUs between local boards and VR and other WIOA programs that are required under WIOA did not document roles and responsibilities for serving employers. We reviewed one MOU for each of the three states with which we conducted in-depth interviews. According to state officials, these MOUs are typical of those used across all local areas in their states. While the local area MOUs we reviewed encourage greater collaboration across workforce programs and describe specific procedures for cross referrals and cost sharing, they do not delineate roles and responsibilities for the employer-facing staff of the various workforce programs to collaborate on working with employers.[38]

One possible negative effect of not having clear, documented roles and responsibilities is the potential for duplicative services provided to employers. VR agencies in our survey reported that they experienced challenges finding single points of contact for employers, with 46 of 73 VR agencies reporting that it is moderately to extremely difficult to do so. In our in-depth interviews, all three states cited the importance of coordination to serve employers. Officials from two states said that their agencies are issuing

---

[36] GAO-12-1022.

[37] None of the agencies that serve only blind or visually impaired individuals reported that they document roles and responsibilities with other workforce programs for serving employers. However, NCSAB officials told us that things have evolved since the time that we administered the survey, and that agencies that serve the blind increasingly are reporting being invited to establish and document those roles.

[38] For example, one AJC official described a delineation of roles whereby VR staff would inform AJC staff about a possible employment opportunity for a VR client, and the AJC staff would reach out to the employer on behalf of that client. The handoff would then be discussed at a regular partner meeting to avoid duplicative outreach.

guidance to help local areas in this regard; officials from the third state said that their agency is developing a client management system to document a single point of contact for businesses, and thereby lessen duplication of efforts. Furthermore, one state VR official told us that without written documentation of roles and responsibilities, she was unsure whether she and the other WIOA program staff would be on the same page to efficiently and effectively address the employment needs of an employer moving to the state.

Employers we spoke with also cited challenges. Employers in one of our employer discussion groups said they were unsure how to navigate the disparate information they received from different workforce programs on the hiring of people with disabilities. Another employer reported that it is not clear that the various agencies working on disability employment are communicating and coordinating effectively.

Education and DOL have provided some technical assistance to states on how to coordinate to serve employers, but have not provided specific examples of how to document roles and responsibilities for coordination across workforce programs in local MOUs. In November 2017, DOL convened a cohort to discuss how to coordinate business services across workforce partners, and in June 2018, made available a webinar to all workforce partners on progress cohort states have made and challenges to integrated business service delivery. DOL noted in training materials for the cohort that roles and responsibilities related to working with employers should be understood and embraced by all partners. However, the template MOUs that Education and DOL made available to the states and local areas do not suggest or include sample language for documenting the roles and responsibilities of each workforce program in serving employers. Having documentation of roles would ensure that responsibilities are clearly delineated and would help prevent duplicative or haphazard outreach to employers.

WIOA specifically requires local boards to include information about cross referrals in their MOUs, but it does not require documentation of roles and responsibilities to serve employers. DOL and Education officials explained that these relationships need to develop over time and stated that they did not think documentation should be required. However, our prior work has found that such documentation helps ensure that coordination can continue even with staff turnover, and may also help the programs articulate a common outcome, leading to more effective collaboration.[39] Documentation may also facilitate more effective leadership in instances such as these where leadership is shared, because local areas may be able to more clearly establish which entity/staff person should take charge in which instances. Fifty-three state VR agencies in our survey reported that it would be helpful to have additional assistance on coordinating with other workforce partners on providing services for employers. Without examples of how to document roles and responsibilities, states may continue to struggle to do this.

Data Sharing or Integration

Relatively few state VR agencies in our survey reported sharing or integrating data, which our prior work has found contributes to the overall resources available to support an interagency collaboration.[40] Fewer than a third (20 of 73) of responding state VR agencies reported sharing data, while more than half (47) reported that data sharing was a work in progress. A much smaller proportion (11 of 73) of responding state VR agencies reported integrating data.[41]

According to one VR official, different data systems across programs make it difficult to coordinate assistance and could result in duplicative effort. A labor official in another state mentioned that the state's VR program would like to access the job postings listed in the AJC system, but the different state agencies have legacy computer systems that do not easily

---

[39] GAO, Workforce Innovation and Opportunity Act: Federal Agencies' Collaboration Generally Reflected Leading Practices, But Could Be Enhanced, GAO-18-171 (Washington, D.C.: February 2018) and GAO-12-1022.

[40] For the purposes of this report, we refer to "data sharing" as sharing of data sets across different programs' systems, and we refer to "data integration" where states are collecting data across programs into one system.

[41] Officials we interviewed from one AJC said that their state is in the process of setting up a universal referral system whereby all the AJC partners can view client case notes in a joint database.

communicate with each other. Further, officials from some state VR agencies, one state labor department, and one AJC cited challenges to data integration and sharing specifically related to confidentiality. For example, one state VR agency explained that in order to share information about a client between two programs, each program must get the client to sign a waiver. The officials stated that waivers are difficult to develop because they are legally binding documents, meaning that lawyers for the partner organizations have to be involved.

DOL and Education officials told us that they are aware that data sharing and integration are a challenge for states and cited efforts to address this challenge. They noted that DOL funds the National Association of State Workforce Agencies' WIOA Information Technology Support Center (WIOA ITSC), which federal and state representatives from WIOA partner programs advise. The Center helps states develop IT systems related to sharing data, integrated service delivery, shared case management, and performance accountability processes. An initiative by a sister organization, the Unemployment Insurance ITSC, is a software suite, Workforce Connect, to help states implement WIOA by integrating Unemployment Insurance, Wagner-Peyser, and workforce IT systems so that they "speak" to each other.

According to the Workforce Connect web site, the suite allows for easy expansion of the modules to new partners in the workforce system, such as adult basic education and VR. The website states that the software suite has been piloted in three states. DOL and Education officials also said that concerns about confidentiality could be addressed in the state-level MOUs that govern the data sharing and potentially in the confidentiality releases that individuals sign. One of Education's VR-focused technical assistance centers has provided a data sharing toolkit and models of how some states are beginning to approach sharing of data. The technical assistance centers told us that, while this is a challenging issue, they expect states to make a lot of progress in the years to come and that they intend to share this progress with other states.

EDUCATION AND DOL HAVE TAKEN STEPS TO MEASURE THE WORKFORCE SYSTEM'S EFFECTIVENESS IN SERVING EMPLOYERS, BUT SOME STATE AGENCIES CITED CONCERNS

In a notice of final rulemaking, Education and DOL proposed a pilot to test three performance measures for assessing the effectiveness of WIOA programs in serving employers.[42] Based on feedback from town halls, workgroups, and comments submitted in response to the notice of proposed rulemaking, Education and DOL selected the proposed measures for further testing. The three proposed performance measures are:[43] (1) *Employer Penetration*—percentage of employers using core WIOA program services out of all employers in the state; (2) *Retention with the Same Employer*—the percentage of participants who are employed with the same employer in the second and fourth quarters after exiting the program; and (3) *Repeat Business Customer*—the percentage of employers who have used WIOA program services more than once in the last 3 years.[44]

Education and DOL are piloting and will evaluate these performance measures to learn more about their validity and reliability.[45] For this nationwide pilot, each state must collect data on two of the three performance measures and report these data annually as a shared outcome across all of the state's core WIOA programs.[46] Education and DOL

---

[42] In this report, we use the term "performance measures" to mean either "indicators for performance" referenced in WIOA or "approaches" referenced in the preamble to the agencies' regulations.

[43] For more information on the three proposed performance measures, see DOL, ETA, *Training and Employment Guidance Letter WIOA NO. 10-16, Change 1- Operating Guidance for WIOA* and Education, RSA, *Technical Assistance Circular 17-01.*

[44] According to a DOL webinar, the Repeat Business Customer proposed performance measure will eventually build into a 3-year cohort. The first year with reportable outcomes, Program Year 2017 (July 2017-June 2018), will be based on repeat business customers for only 1 year. Program Year 2018 will be based on repeat business customers for 2 years. Program Year 2019 and all subsequent years will be based on 3 years' worth of data.

[45] According to Education and DOL officials, the pilot will run from July 2016 to 2020.

[46] As part of the RSA-911 data submitted to Education, VR agencies report whether the client had the same employer during the second quarter and fourth quarter after exit. This data is submitted quarterly and can be used to inform the Retention with the Same Employer performance measure.

explained that having the effectiveness in serving employers performance measures be shared outcomes—meaning that the results from each program are aggregated for the state—will help ensure states and local areas make coordinated efforts to serve employers, because they are being evaluated as such. According to the agencies, due to the lag in data needed for two of three performance measures—Retention with the Same Employer and Repeat Business Customer—states did not report on the three measures as part of their annual WIOA report for program year 2016 (July 2016 to June 2017).[47] According to DOL officials, states will begin reporting pilot outcomes on the three performance measures in October 2018 for program year 2017.

Education and DOL also encouraged states to develop and report on their own "effectiveness in serving employers" performance measures, in addition to reporting on two of the three proposed performance measures, and several states opted to do so. Six of the 74 VR agencies that responded to our survey reported that they are currently developing their own performance measures. For example, one of the six states reported in the survey that it is working with a statistician and gathering input from the business community to develop its own measure of effectiveness in serving employers. In a subsequent communication, an official from this state explained that the state chose to create its own measure to assess the effectiveness of services to employers regardless of the number of services or how often those services were provided. According to this state's survey responses, the state's performance measure aims to assess the correlation between the services provided to the employers and the specific business needs that were satisfactorily met.

During the pilot, DOL is funding a 3-year study to evaluate the feasibility and efficacy of the three performance measures and any additional measures proposed by the states. The evaluation, which began in fall 2017, includes a

[47] According to Education and DOL officials, data for both of these measures were not available in time for the October 2017 reporting deadline because, by definition, the Retention with the Same Employer performance measure is calculated from data reflecting a 1-year period (of individuals employed with the same employer after exiting the VR program) and Repeat Business Customer performance measure is calculated from data reflecting a 3-year period (of employers using WIOA services more than once).

survey of state WIOA administrators, interviews and focus groups with eight states, and a survey of and interviews with select employers. Education and DOL officials said that they will use the results of the survey and interviews, which will run through 2020, to determine if they will choose one performance measure or a suite of measures to assess effectiveness in serving employers. When the evaluation concludes, Education and DOL plan to propose revisions to the current joint regulation to implement their chosen performance measure(s).

In our survey, VR agencies reported varying perspectives on Education and DOL's three proposed performance measures. Of the 62 VR agencies that rated their perspective of the expected effectiveness of the three performance measures, over three fourths rated the Retention with the Same Employer and Repeat Business Customer performance measures as moderately, very, or extremely effective. Just over half of the responding VR agencies (34 out of 62) rated the Employer Penetration rate as moderately, very, or extremely effective (see fig. 5).

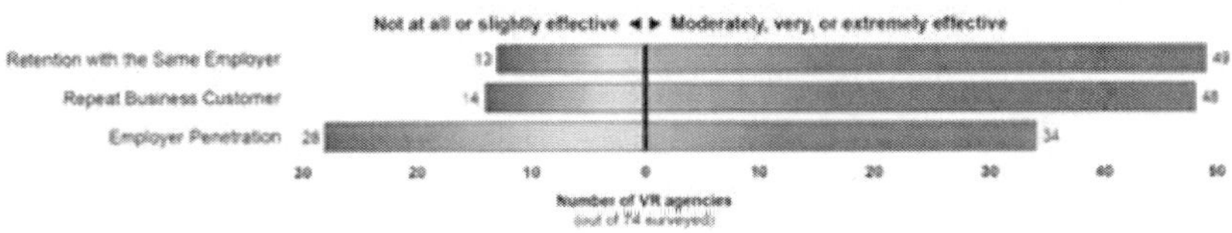

Source: GAO survey of vocational rehabilitation (VR) agencies. | GAO-18-577.

Note: The survey question was: "How effective do you think the following proposed performance measures, if implemented, will be in assessing your state agency's performance in serving employers?" This figure is based on responses from 62 agencies. The other 12 agencies either did not answer the question or responded "don't know."

Figure 5. Expected Effectiveness of the Three Proposed Performance Measures, as Reported by VR Agencies.

Some VR officials cited ways in which the proposed measures may be effective in assessing performance in serving employers. For example, according to one survey respondent, the Retention with the Same Employer measure is effective because it indicates successful placements and the mutual satisfaction of the employer and employee. Another survey respondent said that the Repeat Business Customer measure is the most effective way to measure services to employers because it means that the initial services worked well if employers are returning to use a service again.

However, some state officials expressed specific concerns about the three proposed measures.[48] These concerns raise questions about whether the three performance measures, depending on how they are implemented, would fully reflect several attributes of successful performance measures we previously identified, including clarity, coverage of core program activities, and contextual information.[49]

Clarity

Our prior work has found that successful performance measures are clearly stated and the terms used to calculate the measure have consistent definitions. However, VR agency officials we interviewed in all three states indicated that federal guidance on the proposed performance measures generally lacks clarity because what counts as an employer service is ambiguous. This ambiguity affects the reliability of both the Employer Penetration and Repeat Business Customer proposed performance measures, which rely on states counting the number of employers who are considered to have received a service. Officials we interviewed in one state said that what is meant by or included in terms related to employer service differs not just between Title IV of WIOA, which made changes to the VR program,

---

[48] Because the proposed performance measures are under review by the federal agencies, we are reporting on concerns states shared with us, and we did not independently assess the quality of the performance measures or related guidance.

[49] GAO, *IRS Needs to Further Refine Its Tax Filing Season Performance Measures,* GAO-03-143 (Washington, D.C.: November 22, 2002) and GAO, *DHS Could Better Define How It Plans to Meet Its State and Local Mission and Improve Performance Accountability,* GAO-11-223 (Washington, D.C.: December 16, 2010). These three attributes (clarity, core program activities, and contextual information) are among others identified in GAO-03-143 and GAO-11-223. GAO-03-143 identifies key attributes of successful performance measures and GAO-11-223 identifies key attributes associated with results-oriented management. We developed these attributes based on our previously established criteria from our past work on managing for results.

and other parts of WIOA, but across the 79 VR agencies, such that different VR agencies use terms in different ways.[50] In addition, officials in one of the three states said the subjectivity of when to count employer services may make the proposed Repeat Business Customer and Employer Penetration performance measures more susceptible to data manipulation or error.

Our survey results and interviews suggest that related guidance provided to agencies to-date did not help ensure clarity of these measures. In general, most VR agencies reported in our survey (63 of 74) that additional guidance or technical assistance on the effectiveness in serving employers performance measures would be useful. An official we interviewed in another state said that the state did not receive enough details or specifics provided in what employer services to count towards calculating the performance measures. Officials we interviewed from the third state said that they asked DOL for additional guidance on what services should count toward the proposed Employer Penetration performance measure. While DOL indicated that it was unaware of any confusion with the definition of services for employers, DOL's evaluation of the performance measures will review how different state VR agencies and programs define employer services.[51] DOL and Education do not currently plan to issue additional guidance before the evaluation is completed in 2020. However, this official said that DOL would be willing to provide technical assistance if such confusion exists.

Because the proposed performance measures are shared measures that will be aggregated across the core programs, it is especially important to be clear about what is counted as an employer service. Inconsistency in how core WIOA programs and different levels of government interpret terms related to services to employers could result in confusing or misleading outcomes and may not provide an accurate picture of performance for state and federal officials.

---

[50] The officials mentioned, for example, that the term "worker recruitment" may mean slightly different things under VR versus under other parts of WIOA.

[51] The Statement of Work for the DOL-funded evaluation stated that DOL seeks information about how states, local areas, and federal agencies define "services to employers" and how employer services differ across core WIOA programs, within and across locations and government entities.

Core Program Activities

We previously reported that successful performance measures cover core program activities. However, some states expressed concerns that the proposed performance measures may not sufficiently cover the VR program's core activities. WIOA emphasizes VR agencies' ability to provide education, training, and other services to employers. VR agencies focus on establishing long-term relationships with employers with the goal of placing VR clients with those employers over an extended period of time. One state VR agency official told us that because of barriers to employment facing people with disabilities, these long-term relationships with employers are especially important.[52] In two of the three discussion groups, VR agency officials said that the proposed Employer Penetration performance measure emphasizes the quantity of interactions with employers, which does not necessarily reflect the efforts of VR agencies, which tend to focus on high-quality relationships with fewer employers. In addition, in one of the three discussion groups, VR agency officials said that the proposed performance measures do not adequately capture VR agencies' outreach efforts to employers. One state VR agency official we interviewed noted that placing individuals with disabilities into the right job may take months or sometimes years due to the need to find and mold the job to that person's capabilities. In contrast, this official noted that the other WIOA programs may not have the same challenges and may more easily mold the person into a given job.

Since these performance measures are being piloted as shared measures across the core WIOA programs, including VR, it may be challenging to align all of the core WIOA programs' core program activities with the proposed performance measures. However, to the extent that the proposed performance measures do not sufficiently capture or reflect core VR program activities, they may not fully incentivize activities that are consistent with the VR program's mission.

---

[52] As noted previously, studies have found that, relative to those without disabilities, people with disabilities may face barriers to employment because of employer perceptions and the cost of accommodations.

Contextual Information

We previously reported that performance reporting systems should include contextual or explanatory information to, for example, help clarify aspects of performance that are difficult to quantify. However, some states cited concerns that the proposed performance measures may not account for factors that are outside of VR agencies' control. For example, some states suggested that the performance measures may not account for the business environment. Specifically, VR agency officials in all three discussion groups stated the concern that the proposed Repeat Business Customer performance measure may not reflect the effectiveness of VR agencies' performance because they tend to also serve a lot of small companies that may not need services often. According to VR officials in one state, two-thirds of VR clients' job placements are with small companies because they tend to be more flexible about adapting jobs to VR client's abilities. Meanwhile, a VR official in one discussion group stated that the other WIOA programs would not be as concerned as VR agencies about the effect of small companies on the proposed Repeat Business Customer performance measure because the other WIOA programs serve larger companies that have greater potential for mass hiring.

WIOA also requires that Education and DOL establish an objective statistical model for adjusting performance goals for WIOA programs that factor in economic conditions, such as unemployment rates and job losses or gains, and participant characteristics, including work history, educational attainment, and disability status.[53] While WIOA specifies that the statistical adjustment model will factor in economic conditions such as the unemployment rate in the state, it does not specify that the model reflect the

[53] According to DOL's Training and Employment Guidance Letter 09-17, before the start of each program year, the Secretaries of Labor and Education negotiate with each state to establish a target level of performance for each of the six indicators for that state. The negotiated levels of performance are revised at the end of each year using a statistical adjustment model. According to DOL, the model is a key factor to be used to arrive at agreement on the negotiated state performance levels. The initial statistical adjustment model was developed based on data reported against the Workforce Investment Act of 1998 (WIA) performance measures, which are used as a proxy for WIOA data. The statistical adjustment model will be updated and refined as WIOA outcome data become available.

proportion of small businesses in the state. Officials we interviewed in two of three state VR agencies said that incorporating data on the percentage of small businesses in a state into the statistical adjustment model would be helpful in establishing the proposed Repeat Business Customer performance measure.[54] In finalizing performance measures, if Education and DOL consider factors outside of VR agencies' control (such as the percentage of small businesses in the state), the federal agencies may be better able to fully assess a VR agency's performance, or distinguish it from uncontrollable factors that contribute to a particular result.

CONCLUSION

WIOA has spurred VR agencies to focus more on working with employers and placing clients in mainstream employment. Still, VR agencies face challenges to fully realizing these priorities, and Education has a role to play in helping VR agencies address those challenges. For example, according to employers, VR agencies are challenged to meet their needs for on-demand training. With further assistance from Education on alternative training formats, VR agencies may identify more opportunities to educate front-line managers on disability issues and thereby change perceptions of people with disabilities and promote hiring and retention. VR agencies also reported confusion or inconsistent approaches in the areas of promoting career advancement and mainstream employment. To the extent that Education provides greater access to information about when career advancement services may be provided to employed individuals, VR agencies may better understand the discretion they have to help individuals with disabilities move up the career ladder. In addition, with more complete information from Education about when and how to assess employment settings to determine if they are integrated, VR agencies may be more likely to pursue consistent approaches in this area, including potentially identifying

[54] An official in the third state agency told us the usefulness of incorporating this factor in the statistical model would depend on several factors, such as how small business is defined (i.e., how many employees).

more AbilityOne jobs that are integrated, consistent with federal law and regulations.

Likewise, Education and DOL have roles to play in further enhancing collaboration between VR and other workforce programs, and in addressing VR concerns related to assessing how the workforce system serves employers. Unless Education and DOL provide sample language for states and local areas on how to document roles and responsibilities for serving employers, workforce programs may not independently build such language into their written agreements, thereby limiting their ability to take a coordinated approach. This can result in frustration on the part of employers and wasted time on the part of workforce staff, and in the worst cases, jeopardize the public workforce system's valuable relationship with employers and the potential for placement of clients. Also, by taking into account state VR agencies' concerns when finalizing the performance measures for effectiveness in serving employers, Education and DOL are more likely to implement measures that: have clear definitions that help ensure data reliability; are linked to core VR program activities, which could incentivize activities that support the VR program's population and mission; and reflect key contextual factors outside of VR agency control, thereby ensuring clearer performance data and realistic performance targets.

Recommendations for Executive Action

We are making seven recommendations; five are to Education and two are to DOL. Specifically:

The Commissioner of Education's Rehabilitation Services Administration should work with state VR agencies to determine whether and what additional information and assistance VR agencies may find helpful regarding on-demand training, such as online videos, to employers on disability issues. (Recommendation 1)

The Commissioner of Education's Rehabilitation Services Administration should work with state VR agencies to determine how to most effectively disseminate information about the circumstances in which individuals who are employed may be eligible for career advancement services. (Recommendation 2)

The Commissioner of Education's Rehabilitation Services Administration should work with state VR agencies to develop more complete information on when and how VR agencies should assess employment settings, including settings supported by the AbilityOne program, to determine if they meet the definition of competitive integrated employment. (Recommendation 3)

The Commissioner of Education's Rehabilitation Services Administration should encourage local areas to clarify and document the roles and responsibilities of partner agencies in working with employers and provide sample language of how local areas may document roles and responsibilities in their MOUs. (Recommendation 4)

The Commissioner of Education's Rehabilitation Services Administration should, in setting the employer performance measurement approaches with DOL after the pilot is concluded, take into account VR agencies' concerns and key attributes of successful performance measures, including clarity in what is meant by employer services, coverage of the VR agencies' core program activities, and consideration of factors outside of VR agencies' control. (Recommendation 5)

The Assistant Secretary of DOL's Employment and Training Administration should encourage local areas to clarify and document the roles and responsibilities of partner agencies in working with employers and provide sample language of how local areas may document roles and responsibilities in their MOUs. (Recommendation 6)

The Assistant Secretary of DOL's Employment and Training Administration should, in setting the employer performance measurement approaches with Education after the pilot is concluded, take into account VR agencies' concerns and key attributes of successful performance measures, including clarity in what is meant by employer services, coverage of the VR agencies' core program activities, and consideration of factors outside of VR agencies' control. (Recommendation 7)

AGENCY COMMENTS AND OUR EVALUATION

We provided a draft of this chapter to Education and DOL for their review and comment, and provided relevant excerpts to the U.S. AbilityOne Commission. See appendix III for Education's comments and appendix IV for DOL's comments.

For the five recommendations aimed at Education, Education neither agreed nor disagreed. In its comments, Education emphasized that state VR agencies have the primary responsibility for determining how best to meet employers' needs, promote mainstream employment, and collaborate with other workforce programs in their states. We agree that it is appropriate for the state VR agencies to develop policies and approaches in all of these areas to fit the needs of their individual and employer clients. At the same time, Education acknowledged that it can play a role in helping state agencies and noted that it will take or consider taking additional steps to assist state agencies in each area where we made recommendations. Specifically:

- With regard to recommendation 1, Education recognized the importance of providing information and technical assistance to state VR agencies to help them serve employers, while stressing that it is a state matter how to best meet the training needs of employers. Education suggested that the recommendation emphasize the need to work with states to determine what information they would find helpful, and we clarified the recommendation accordingly.
- With regard to recommendation 2, Education recognized the importance of expanding career advancement opportunities for individuals with disabilities in accordance with the Rehabilitation Act as amended by WIOA. At the same time, Education said it is up to states to determine how to most effectively disseminate information about their services. Education noted it will continue to work with state VR agencies to determine what additional information may be necessary about the circumstances in which individuals who are employed may be eligible for career advancement services.

- With regard to recommendation 3, Education said that it is a state matter to determine whether an employment location qualifies as an "integrated setting" for the purpose of the VR program, and that it is not Education's role to inform states as to when and how to make such determinations. Nevertheless, Education said it will continue to work with the states to determine if additional information would help them assess employment locations.
- With regard to recommendation 4, Education said it believes that state workforce development agencies are in the best position to lead employer engagement efforts, but will continue to collaborate with other federal partners to provide technical assistance to states in this area, including examples of state- and local-level collaboration on employer engagement.
- With regard to recommendation 5, Education said it will work with DOL to ensure that state VR agencies' concerns are considered when the performance measure for effectiveness in serving employers is finalized.

After Education provided its formal response, the Assistant Secretary, Office of Special Education and Rehabilitative Services, clarified in an email that the agency disagreed with recommendations 1, 2, and 3; neither agreed nor disagreed with recommendation 4; and agreed with recommendation 5.

DOL agreed with recommendations 6 and 7. For recommendation 6, DOL said that local workforce boards and one-stop partners are in the best position to lead employer engagement, but that it will collaborate with federal partners in providing related technical assistance. For recommendation 7, DOL said it will coordinate with Education to ensure state VR agencies' concerns are considered in defining the performance measure.

In addition, Education, DOL, and the U.S. AbilityOne Commission provided technical comments, which we incorporated as appropriate.

As agreed with your office, unless you publicly announce the contents of this chapter earlier, we plan no further distribution until 30 days from the report date. At that time, we will send copies of this chapter to the appropriate congressional committees, the Secretary of the Department of Education, the Secretary of the Department of Labor, the Executive Director of the U.S. AbilityOne Commission, and other interested parties.

Sincerely yours,

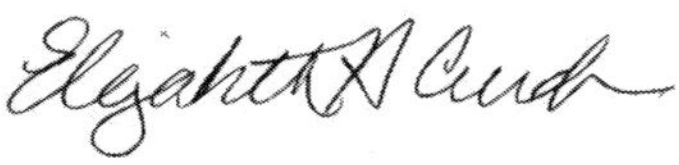

Elizabeth H. Curda, Director
Education, Workforce, and Income Security Issues

APPENDIX I: OBJECTIVES, SCOPE, AND METHODOLOGY

This chapter to examines (1) the steps vocational rehabilitation (VR) agencies have taken under the Workforce Innovation and Opportunity Act (WIOA) to work with employers and place individuals in mainstream employment, and the extent which the Department of Education (Education) has helped them address any challenges; (2) how VR agencies have coordinated with other workforce programs to effectively serve individual clients and employers, and the extent to which federal agencies have addressed any challenges; and (3) the extent to which Education and the Department of Labor (DOL) have measured VR agencies' efforts to serve employers under WIOA.

We took the following steps to address all three objectives. We reviewed pertinent federal laws and regulations. We reviewed guidance disseminated by Education and DOL, such as on the definition of competitive integrated employment, data matching across WIOA programs for performance reporting, and WIOA unified and combined state plans, as well as technical assistance documents generated by the technical assistance centers, such as toolkits on the memorandum of understanding with the local workforce development board and on data sharing agreements. We interviewed officials from Education, including the Rehabilitation Services Administration; DOL, including the Employment and Training

Administration; technical assistance centers; the Council of State Administrators of Vocational Rehabilitation (CSAVR); the National Council of State Agencies for the Blind; the National Association of Workforce Boards; the U.S. AbilityOne Commission; SourceAmerica; National Industries for the Blind; National Council on Independent Living; and Respect Ability. To further understand how VR agencies are promoting mainstream employment, we obtained and reviewed data from the U.S. AbilityOne Commission, including the number of individuals in AbilityOne employment during fiscal year 2016 and their average wages. We assessed the reliability of these data by interviewing U.S. AbilityOne Commission officials, and found the data to be sufficiently reliable for our reporting purposes.

Survey of VR Agencies

To address all three objectives, we administered a web-based survey questionnaire to the directors of all 79 state VR agencies. Data collection began in October 2017 and ended in December 2017. We made follow-up email and telephone contacts throughout this period to encourage response. We received 74 survey responses (94 percent of the population), which describe the steps those agencies have taken to provide services to employers as well as the challenges they report facing. The survey, for example, asked how services to employers changed since the enactment of WIOA and ways VR agencies are coordinating with the other WIOA programs. We also asked about the degree of difficulty they have experienced in potentially challenging areas, such as meeting the demands of businesses and coordinating with the other WIOA programs on contacting businesses. To reduce the overall survey burden on these respondents, we also asked questions to inform a related GAO engagement on pre-employment transition services for youth.

We took steps to minimize the potential errors that the practical difficulties of conducting any survey may introduce. Because we selected the entire population of VR agencies into our survey, our estimates are not subject to sampling error. Nonresponse error can result when a survey fails to capture information from all cases sampled, or in this case, the population. Nonresponse reduces the precision of estimates due to the smaller number of observations, and can introduce bias if those not responding, in the aggregate, would have given materially different answers to a question compared to those who did respond. The known characteristics of the five agencies that did not respond indicate that they are smaller, on average, than those who did respond, in terms of their eligible service populations, numbers served, and grant totals. These three characteristics may or may not be related to the nature of agency answers to some questions. However, the nonresponding agencies did not materially differ from responding agencies across the fourth known characteristic—the percentage of their state populations in urban areas. In addition, the totals for each of the first three characteristics—service populations, numbers served, and grant amounts—across the five nonresponding agencies comprised less than one percent of the totals for the population, suggesting a lower possibility of material error in our results from nonresponse of these five smaller agencies. We conducted pretests of the draft questionnaire with three agencies in the population and made revisions to reduce the possibility of measurement error from differences in how questions were interpreted and the sources of information available to respondents. A second, independent analyst checked the accuracy of all computer analyses to minimize the likelihood of errors in data processing.

Discussion Groups with VR Agencies

To address all three objectives, we conducted discussion groups during a national, CSAVR-sponsored conference of VR agencies in November 2017 in Greenville, South Carolina. To recruit participants, we worked with CSAVR to invite VR agencies to our discussion groups. CSAVR included an invitation to our discussion groups in an e-mail sent to all VR agencies before the conference, and encouraged participation during opening remarks at the conference. We also solicited participants through our survey of VR agencies. We conducted follow up calls to survey respondents who indicated an interest in participating in the discussion groups to further encourage participation. Since discussion groups took place in person at the conference, participants did not include VR agencies that did not attend the conference.

We conducted three discussion groups with 9 to 15 participants per group. Discussion group participants consisted of 36 VR agency directors or their designees from 24 separate VR agencies. The questions for the discussion groups included topics on states' experiences in working with employers, coordination with the WIOA workforce programs, technical assistance and guidance from the federal agencies, and perspectives on the performance measures. GAO facilitators conducted the discussion groups.

Interviews with VR and Other Workforce Program Officials in Select States

To address all three objectives, we conducted in-depth phone interviews (and in-person interviews when possible) with state VR agency officials and state labor department officials from three states: Alabama, Arizona, and Maryland. We selected these three states to obtain a mix in terms of the following criteria: state agency organization (the state agency that houses the VR agency), size of the client population using the number of clients that the VR agency served in fiscal year 2014, the percentage of the population living in an urbanized area in the state, whether the state had been recommended to us or not in preliminary interviews as having well developed employer services or collaborative practices across workforce partners, and geographic diversity using DOL's regional office areas (see table 1).

We also interviewed officials at American Job Centers (AJC) in at least one local area in each state. We chose local areas to obtain a mix in the percentage of the population with a disability, percentage of the population in an urbanized area, and labor force participation rate. Based on these criteria, we selected AJC sites from the three states: Demopolis Career Center and Fayette Career Center (Alabama), Coconino Career Center (Arizona), and WorkSource Montgomery (Maryland) (see table 2).

Table1. States Selected for Site Visits or Interviews

State	State agency organization	Number of clients served	Percentage of the population living in an urbanized area[a]	Recommended in preliminary interviews	Geographic diversity
Alabama	Department of Rehabilitation Services	6,653	48.7%	Yes	Region 3– Atlanta
Arizona	Department of Economic Security	2,481	80.1%	No	Region 6– San Francisco
Maryland	State Department of Education	4,307	83.5%	Yes	Region 2– Philadelphia

Source: GAO analysis. | GAO-18-577.

[a] These are 2010 data from the U.S. Census Bureau.

Table 2. Local Areas Selected for Site Visits or Interviews

County and state in which American Job Center is located	American Job Center	Percentage of the population with a disability[a]	Percentage of the population living in an urbanized area[b]	Percentage of the population in the labor force[a]
Fayette and Marengo Counties, Alabama	Fayette Career Center and Demopolis Career Center	23.7%–27.5%	0.0%	48.2%–49.8%
Coconino County, Arizona	Coconino Career Center	11.5%	53.5%	63.9%
Montgomery County, Maryland	WorkSource Montgomery	7.9%	97.1%	71.8%

Source: GAO analysis. | GAO-18-577.

[a] The source of these data are American Community Survey 5-Year Estimates 2012–2016.

[b] These are 2010 data from the U.S. Census Bureau.

Interview question topics included states' efforts to provide services to employers since the enactment of WIOA, VR agencies and the other WIOA programs efforts to coordinate services to individuals and employers, and perspectives on the effectiveness of the performance measures. Since we interviewed officials in only three states, we cannot conclude that their experiences are representative of those nationwide.

Discussion Groups with Employers

To address objectives one and two and understand employers' perspective on the VR program, we conducted discussion groups with employers that have had some interaction with the VR program. We held four discussion groups: one each in Birmingham, Alabama, and King of Prussia, Pennsylvania, and two in Oakland, California. We spoke with representatives of 29 employers total across the three sites: 10 in Alabama, 5 in Pennsylvania, and 14 in California.[1] We spoke with private and public sector employers. Our discussion questions for employers covered topics including how employers became aware of VR services, why employers chose to use VR services, what VR services were used, and how well VR services met employers' needs.

Our discussions were held in conjunction with employer outreach events conducted by CSAVR. As part of each event, we recruited employers for our discussion groups with the help of the state VR agency. In Alabama, according to a state official, the VR agency invited 50 employers that were at least aware of the VR program to participate in the CSAVR event; 20 employers accepted the invitation; and among these the 10 employers that had a working relationship with the VR agency were invited to participate in the GAO discussion group. In Pennsylvania, according to state officials, about 60 employer representatives were invited to participate in the GAO discussion group, including all members of a business group active in disability issues and all employer representatives registered to attend the

---

[1] In California, some employers had representatives in both of the discussion groups we held.

employer outreach event; the employer representatives who chose to speak with GAO had all worked with the VR agency in some way. In California, according to a state official, the VR agency invited to the event all employers that had worked with VR and were within reasonable traveling distance of Oakland; and the GAO discussion groups included all employers who accepted the invitation and participated in the event. The results of our discussion groups cannot be generalized to employers more broadly.

Criteria Applied

To assess Education's efforts to address VR agencies' challenges with meeting employer needs and promoting mainstream employment, we applied standards for internal control in the federal government.[2] Specifically, we applied principle 15 related to communicating with external parties. In addition, we relied on a guide for assessing federal agencies' training and development efforts that we previously developed, particularly the criteria related to how agencies compare the merits of different mechanisms for delivering training.[3]

To assess coordination among VR agencies and other workforce programs, we applied key considerations for implementing interagency collaborative mechanisms that we have previously identified.[4] In our prior work, we identified seven features of effective interagency collaboration, and in this chapter we describe the extent to which collaboration among workforce programs exhibits these features.

Finally, in examining state VR agencies' concerns with pilot performance measures for effectiveness in serving employers, we considered how these concerns related to key attributes of effective

---

[2] GAO, Standards for Internal Control in the Federal Government, GAO-14-704G (Washington, D.C.: September 2014).

[3] GAO, Human Capital: A Guide for Assessing Strategic Training and Development Efforts in the Federal Government, GAO-04-546G (Washington, D.C.: March 2004).

[4] GAO, Managing for Results: Key Considerations for Implementing Interagency Collaborative Mechanisms, GAO-12-1022 (Washington, D.C.: Sept. 27, 2012).

performance measures that we have previously identified.[5] In our prior work we have identified more than 10 such attributes, and in this work we tied agencies' concerns to three attributes related to clarity, core program activities, and contextual information.

APPENDIX II: THE WORKFORCE SYSTEM

Table 3 describes the six WIOA core programs administered by DOL and Education.

Table 3. Workforce Innovation and Opportunity Act (WIOA) Core Programs

Administered by Department of Labor (DOL)[a]	
Title I Adult	Provides training and services, such as occupational skills training, career counseling, and job searches, to adults ages 18 or older (recipients of public assistance, other low-income individuals, and individuals who are basic skills deficient receive priority for certain services)
Title I Dislocated Worker	Provides the same services as the Title I Adult program for those who, generally, among other criteria, anticipate or have been terminated or laid-off or who were self-employed
Title I Youth	Provides various services, including educational supports, occupational skills training, counseling, and paid and unpaid work experiences, generally to lowincome youth who are facing one or more barriers to employment
Wagner-Peyser Employment Services	Provides employment services, including job searches and placement assistance, and referrals to employers (veterans receive priority for certain services and individuals with disabilities, migrant and seasonal farmworkers, ex-offenders, and several other populations receive specialized services)
Adult Education and Family Literacy Act	Generally assists adults (and youth age 16 and older who are not enrolled or required to be enrolled in secondary school) in becoming literate or achieving proficiency in English, obtaining the knowledge and skills necessary for employment and self-sufficiency and to assist in their children's educational development, and completing a secondary school education

[5] GAO, Information Sharing: DHS Could Better Define How It Plans to Meet Its State and Local Mission and Improve Performance Accountability, GAO-11-223 (Washington, D.C.: Dec.16, 2010). GAO, Tax Administration: IRS Needs to Further Refine Its Tax Filing Season Performance Measures, GAO-03-143 (Washington, D.C.: Nov. 22, 2002).

Administered by Department of Education (Education)[b]	
State Vocational Rehabilitation Services	Provides services such as counseling, job training, and job search assistance, related to the employment of people with disabilities

Source: GAO-16-287 and GAO analysis of federal law and agency information | GAO-18-577.

[a] DOL's Employment and Training Administration (ETA) administers these programs and oversees their implementation, which is carried out by state workforce agencies and local workforce development boards. The local board selects the entities that will operate American Job Centers (formerly called one-stop centers) to provide services.

[b] Education's Office of Career, Technical, and Adult Education (OCTAE) provides grants to states, which in turn distribute most of the federal funds to local adult education providers. The local provider network includes local educational agencies, community colleges, community-based organizations, and volunteer literacy organizations. Education's Rehabilitation Services Administration (RSA) provides grants to states to administer the Vocational Rehabilitation program. Many states have separate agencies serving blind or visually impaired individuals in addition to agencies that serve all other individuals with disabilities. In addition, states vary in terms of the organizational positioning of the program, with the program being housed in education, workforce, social service, or disability program agencies, or elsewhere.

APPENDIX III: COMMENTS FROM THE DEPARTMENT OF EDUCATION

UNITED STATES DEPARTMENT OF EDUCATION
OFFICE OF SPECIAL EDUCATION AND REHABILITATIVE SERVICES

THE ASSISTANT SECRETARY

JUL 19 2018

Elizabeth H. Curda
Director
Education, Workforce and
Income Security Issues
U.S. Government Accountability Office
441 G Street, NW
Washington, DC 20548

Dear Ms. Curda:

I am writing in response to the recommendations made in the U.S. Government Accountability Office (GAO) draft report, "Vocational Rehabilitation: Additional Federal Information Could Help States Serve Employers and Find Jobs for People with Disabilities" (GAO-18-577). We appreciate the opportunity to comment on the draft report on behalf of the U.S. Department of Education (Department).

Vocational rehabilitation (VR) has historically been a client-centered program and process. As GAO notes, the Workforce Innovation and Opportunity Act (WIOA) included changes to the Rehabilitation Act of 1973 (Rehabilitation Act) increasing the focus on employers and services to employers to facilitate the achievement of competitive integrated employment by individuals with disabilities. We appreciate GAO's review of the employer aspects of the vocational rehabilitation process, and related issues of employment settings, career advancement and program performance measures under WIOA.

The draft report includes seven recommendations; five made to the Department and two to the U.S. Department of Labor. We are providing our responses to the five recommendations made to the Department. We note that the two recommendations made to the Department of Labor are similar and complementary to the fourth and fifth recommendations made to the Department of Education, and we intend to work cooperatively with the Department of Labor in resolving them.

Recommendation 1: *The Commissioner of Education's Rehabilitation Services Administration should provide information and assistance to VR agencies to help them offer on-demand training, such as online videos, to employers on disability issues.*

Response: The Department recognizes the importance of providing information and technical assistance to State VR agencies to help them work effectively with employers. However, the Department believes strongly that it is a State matter as to how VR agencies can best meet the training and technical assistance needs of employers in their States, whether it be on-demand or in-person. To that end, the Department's Rehabilitation Services Administration (RSA) suggests that this recommendation be revised to read: *The Commissioner of Education's Rehabilitation Services Administration should work with State VR agencies to determine whether and what information and assistance VR agencies may find helpful regarding offering on-demand training, such as online videos, to employers on disability issues.*

Furthermore, we note that RSA has provided training and technical assistance to the State VR agencies regarding their responsibilities under the Rehabilitation Act, as amended by WIOA, to work with and provide technical assistance to employers, particularly those interested in hiring individuals with disabilities. In so doing, RSA funded the Job Driven Vocational Rehabilitation Technical Assistance Center, now in its no-cost extension year, to provide such technical assistance. The Department will work with State VR agencies to assess their technical assistance and training needs on disability issues for employers.

Recommendation 2: *The Commissioner of Education's Rehabilitation Services Administration should work with state VR agencies to determine how to most effectively disseminate information about the circumstances in which individuals who are employed may be eligible for career advancement services.*

Response: The Department recognizes the importance of expanding career advancement opportunities for individuals with disabilities in accordance with the Rehabilitation Act as amended by WIOA. The preamble to the VR regulations published at 81 FR 55630, 55672 and 55677 (August 19, 2016) discusses eligibility for the VR program for the purpose of career advancement and the availability of VR services, such as advanced training, to assist eligible individuals to advance in their employment. These concepts also were discussed at several national meetings (e.g., meetings of the Council of State Administrators of Vocational Rehabilitation). However, it is important to note that nothing in the Rehabilitation Act, prior to the amendments made by WIOA, prohibited VR agencies from determining an individual's eligibility on the basis of his or her desire to advance in employment. It is the Department's longstanding position that an individual with a disability is eligible for VR services if he or she requires VR services to advance in employment. The Department will continue to work with State VR agencies to determine if additional information may be necessary about the circumstances in which individuals who are employed may be eligible for career advancement services. The Department believes strongly that it is a State matter for VR agencies to determine how to most effectively disseminate information about the services they provide.

Recommendation 3: *The Commissioner of Education's Rehabilitation Services Administration should work with state VR agencies to develop more complete information on when and how VR agencies should assess employment settings, including settings supported by the AbilityOne program, to determine if they meet the definition of competitive integrated employment.*

Response: The Department has made it clear for many years, including in the preamble to the Final Regulations published at 81 FR 55630, that determinations of whether an employment location would be considered an "integrated setting," for purposes of the VR program, is a matter of State determination. We do not believe it is the Department's role to inform the States as to when and how to make such determinations. The VR agencies are privy to all facts of any given employment location and are in the best position to make such decisions whenever questions arise. However, the Department will continue to work with State VR agencies to determine if further information is needed regarding when and how State VR agencies should assess

employment settings to determine whether such settings meet the definition of competitive integrated employment.

Recommendation 4: *The Commissioner of Education's Rehabilitation Services Administration should encourage local areas to clarify and document the roles and responsibilities of partner agencies in working with employers and provide sample language of how local areas may document roles and responsibilities in their MOUs.*

Response: The Department believes that State workforce development agencies, as one-stop partners who collaborate with local workforce development boards and chief elected officials, are in the best position to lead employer engagement at the local level. The conceptual framework for WIOA is structured around local control and flexibility. The Department's RSA, in partnership with the Department of Labor's Employment and Training Administration and the Department's Office of Career, Technical and Adult Education, has provided extensive joint guidance and technical assistance to local areas related to the one-stop service delivery system, including a Sample MOU Toolkit. RSA will continue to collaborate with its Federal partners in delivering technical assistance that reinforces the role of State and local partners, including examples of how other State and local partners have collaborated on employer engagement given the flexibility that WIOA provides.

Recommendation 5: *The Commissioner of Education's Rehabilitation Services Administration should, in setting the employer performance measurement approaches with DOL after the pilot is concluded, take into account VR agencies' concerns and key attributes of successful performance measures, including clarity in what is meant by employer services, coverage of the VR agencies' core program activities, and consideration of factors outside of VR agencies' control.*

Response: The Department will coordinate with the Department of Labor's Employment and Training Administration to ensure that State VR agencies' concerns are considered in determining the performance measures regarding the "Effectiveness in Serving Employers" performance measure. The determination also will be informed by the results of the evaluation of this performance measure, scheduled to be available in 2020.

The Department appreciates the opportunity to review the draft report and comment on the recommendations. We also are enclosing technical comments for your consideration.

Sincerely,

Johnny W. Collett

Appendix IV: Comments from the Department of Labor

U.S. Department of Labor

Employment and Training Administration
200 Constitution Avenue, N.W.
Washington, D.C. 20210

Elizabeth Curda
Director
Education, Workforce, and Income Security Issues
U.S. Government Accountability Office
441 G Street, N.W.
Washington, D.C. 20548

Dear Ms. Curda:

Thank you for the opportunity to review and comment on the Government Accountability Office's (GAO) draft report titled, *Vocational Rehabilitation: Additional Federal Information Could Help States Serve Employers and Find Jobs for People with Disabilities* (GAO-18-577, job code 102179). We understand that GAO performed this work pursuant to its authority under 31 U.S.C. 717 after receiving a request from Ranking Member Patty Murray of the Senate Committee on Health, Education, Labor, and Pensions.

The Department of Labor (Department) appreciates GAO's work to provide information and to document the progress made and the remaining challenges in implementing the Workforce Innovation and Opportunity Act (WIOA).

The Department has worked closely with the Department of Education (ED) for several years to identify our grantees' greatest needs and to jointly develop and disseminate technical assistance and guidance as necessary. The Department will continue to work with ED to consider how best to support integrated business services at the local level, through flexibilities and technical assistance. The Department agrees with both recommendations from GAO, 6 and 7, which were targeted toward the Department of Labor.

The Department agrees with GAO Recommendation 6, that the Employment and Training Administration (ETA) should encourage local areas to clarify and document the roles and responsibilities of partner agencies in their Memoranda of Understanding. However, it recognizes that local workforce development boards and local one-stop partners are in the best position to lead employer engagement at the local level. The Department, in partnership with the Department of Education, has provided extensive joint guidance and technical assistance to local areas related to the one-stop service delivery system, including a Sample MOU Toolkit. The Department will continue to collaborate with its Federal partners in delivering technical assistance that reinforces that WIOA provides flexibility in how states and local partners engage employers. This includes examples of how other state and local partners have collaborated on employer engagement.

Regarding the *Effectiveness in Serving Employers* performance measure definition, the Department concurs with GAO Recommendation 7. The Department will coordinate with Education's Rehabilitation Services Administration (RSA) to ensure that Vocational Rehabilitation (VR) agencies' concerns are considered in defining this performance measure.

The determination of the definition also will be informed by the results of the evaluation of this performance measure, due in 2020.

Thank you for the opportunity to respond.

Sincerely,

Rosemary Lahasky
Acting Assistant Secretary for Employment and Training
U.S. Department of Labor

APPENDIX V: STAFF ACKNOWLEDGEMENTS

In addition to Elizabeth H. Curda, Michele Grgich (Assistant Director); Lorin Obler (Analyst-In-Charge); Laurie Chin; Holly Dye; and Srinidhi Vijaykumar made key contributions to this chapter. Also contributing to this chapter were James Bennett, Shannon Finnegan, Alex Galuten, Lauren Gilbertson, Ben Licht, Sheila McCoy, Sam Portnow, Carl Ramirez, Monica Savoy, Almeta Spencer, and Alexandra Squitieri.

INDEX

D

F

G

H

I

J

K

L

M

N

O

P

R

S

T

U

V

W

Y

Special Education: Developments, Teaching Strategies and Parental Involvement

Editor: Shaun Bowman

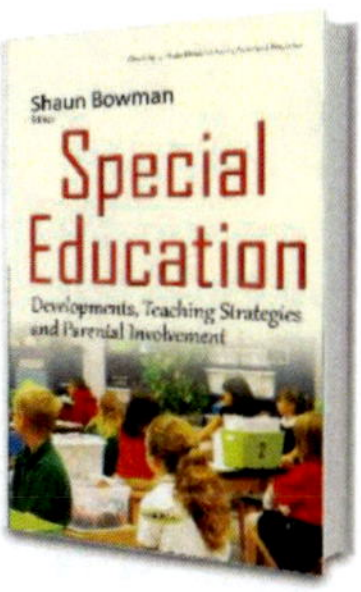

Series: Disability and the Disabled-Issues, Laws and

Book Description: The authors of this book discuss the latest developments in special education research. The chapters included examine the three main components of "sense of coherence," all of which are involved in the long-term outcome of people in special education, and the development and evaluation of competency-based teacher training programs in the field of special education.

Hardcover ISBN: 978-1-63483-875-7
Retail Price: $192

Physical Disabilities: Perspectives, Risk Factors and Quality of Life

Editor: Lawrence Mitchell

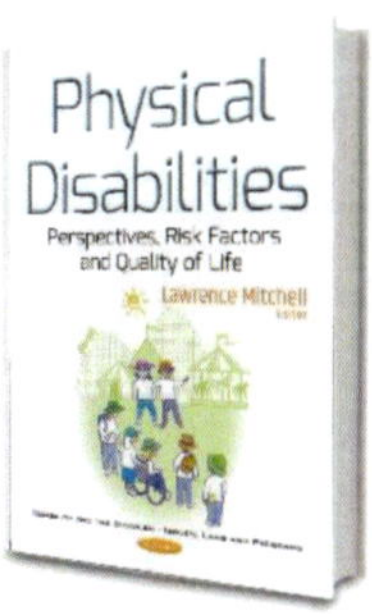

Series: Disability and the Disabled – Issues, Laws and Programs, Physical Medicine and Rehabilitation

Book Description: Physical disabilities are impairments which limit an individual's physical function. This book reviews risk factors and the affect physical disabilities have on quality of life.

Softcover ISBN: 978-1-53610-857-6
Retail Price: $82